The Palgrave Lacan Series

Series Editors
Calum Neill
School of Applied Sciences
Edinburgh Napier University
Edinburgh, UK

Derek Hook
Duquesne University
Pittsburgh, USA

Jacques Lacan is one of the most important and influential thinkers of the 20th century. The reach of this influence continues to grow as we settle into the 21st century, the resonance of Lacan's thought arguably only beginning now to be properly felt, both in terms of its application to clinical matters and in its application to a range of human activities and interests. The Palgrave Lacan Series is a book series for the best new writing in the Lacanian field, giving voice to the leading writers of a new generation of Lacanian thought. The series will comprise original monographs and thematic, multi-authored collections. The books in the series will explore aspects of Lacan's theory from new perspectives and with original insights. There will be books focused on particular areas of or issues in clinical work. There will be books focused on applying Lacanian theory to areas and issues beyond the clinic, to matters of society, politics, the arts and culture. Each book, whatever its particular concern, will work to expand our understanding of Lacan's theory and its value in the 21st century.

More information about this series at
http://www.palgrave.com/gp/series/15116

Raul Moncayo

Knowing, Not-Knowing, and Jouissance

Levels, Symbols, and Codes of Experience in Psychoanalysis

palgrave
macmillan

Raul Moncayo
Berkeley, CA, USA

The Palgrave Lacan Series
ISBN 978-3-030-06769-4 ISBN 978-3-319-94003-8 (eBook)
https://doi.org/10.1007/978-3-319-94003-8

Softcover re-print of the Hardcover 1st edition 2018

Cover illustration: Tim Gainey/Alamy Stock Photo

Printed on acid-free paper

This Palgrave Macmillan imprint is published by the registered company Springer International Publishing AG part of Springer Nature
The registered company address is: Gewerbestrasse 11, 6330 Cham, Switzerland

Preface and Acknowledgements

The ideas in this book emerged from several independent projects that slowly coalesced into a book. Chapter 1 is a follow up to my doctoral dissertation (1984) that entailed a detailed exegesis of Freud's two theories of mind centered around the concept of repression and its cultural implications/foundations. In Chapter 1 wanted to ascertain how some specific theoretical questions/problems raised by Freud in the Metapsychology were or not answered/solved by Lacanian theory. In addition, I wanted to highlight a distinction between awareness and consciousness, found implicit in Freud's theory, and link this concept of awareness to unconscious or un-self-conscious forms of knowing. While I was writing, I was asked to write a review for Bristow's book on Joyce and Lacan and found that what supported Joyce in his writing had some links to the concept of awareness I was searching for in the Metapsychology and beyond. In addition, I reconsider the merits of Freud's energetic and economic point of view in the light of contemporary physics, Lacan's theory of jouissance, post-structuralism's privileging of energetic intensities over representational schemas of meaning, and, finally, the fact that the rest of psychoanalysis (object relations and the interpersonal schools) considers Freud's energetic ideas *passé* and outdated.

Chapter 2 was inspired by an email I received some years ago from a reader who wanted me to read some texts on Darwinian theory and evolutionary psychology. Perhaps their motivation was influenced by Dylan Evans' *in toto* adoption of Darwinism, not long after publishing what to this day is the only dictionary of Lacanian psychoanalysis in English. I read the recommended texts and discovered that biology nowadays considers Darwinism (coupled with evolutionary genetics and the new field of epigenetics) a meta-framework for the biological field. At the same time, evolutionary psychology makes no attempt to address human sexuality within the context of culture and the symbolic order, the way that Freud and Lacan have done with psychoanalysis. In addition, the cultural ideas that emerge from Darwinism represent very outdated, if not downright racist and sexist views about society. Without Freudian theory, Darwinian concepts are not enough to understand how biological instincts function within cultural symbolic orders.

Chapter 3 was written not only to show the inner consistencies between Freud and Lacan's theory of the drive, but also how the accent on the grammatical voice of the drive definitely falls on cultural rather than biological factors, and therefore can be regarded as a rebuke of the criticism that Freud was a pseudo biologist of the mind. A specific example of this is how Lacan transformed Freud's idea that the body imposes a certain demand for work on the Mind (that responds with cultural signifiers and representations), into a social/sexual demand of the subject to be demanded/repressed or seduced by the Other. Mind and Other here occupy similar structural positions.

Chapter 4 was precipitated by a weekly Seminar with Barri Belnap and Greg Farr from the Austen Riggs Center in Massachusetts, where John Muller combined Lacanian psychoanalysis, developmental psychoanalytic psychology, and Peirce's semiotics. Lacan engaged Pierce's work in his Seminar IX on Identification, which was a central focus of my book *The Emptiness of Oedipus*. Muller also knew the late Roberto Harari who was my first mentor in psychoanalysis. This Chapter explores the relations between Semiotic and Symbolic Codes in reference to psychoanalysis. Chapter 5 explores what happens to Freud's structural theory of personality in the light of Lacan's critique of ego psychology, his utilization of the concepts of the ideal ego and ego ideal by way of '*mathemes*', and Lacan's own concepts of the subject/signifier and the subject in/of the Real.

Chapter 6 is an enlarged version of a review/response that was published by the Journal of the Circle for Lacanian Ideology Critique, Vol. 10, 2017 under the editorial guidance of Sigi Jottkandt. The response was precipitated by a paper by S. Brahnam where she worked Lacan's exercises involving probability theory and cybernetics that appear as an addendum to his text on *The Purloined Letter*. As the chapter stands now, it also represents a Lacanian and psychoanalytic commentary on digital and computer culture.

The stimulus for Chapter 7 on Lacan's late *ecrit L'étourdit* came from a joint event on the topic co-sponsored by the Lacanian School and Marcus Coelen, Jamieson Webster, and Patricia Gherovici. For this book in particular, and as a link between Chapters 6 and 7, I expanded a section addressing the mention of mathematics and logic in Lacan's text. This is in response to questions and reviews of a prior book, to critiques of Lacan's use of mathematics, and to delimit the area within which conceptual mathematics may be most useful to psychoanalytic theory.

Chapter 8 emerged from my study of Lacan's *Seminar XIX, … ou pire* where Lacan continues the evolution of his teaching in the direction of the One of the Real that 'ex-sists' 'All-alone' in the place of the absence of a sexual rapport between the sexes. The One All-alone represents a form of benevolent solitude that does not prevent relationships between the sexes nor the sexual act. This is the Lacanian response to the current problems between the sexes and to the failure of the old ideal norm that the fusion of love and sex in marriage could represent a stable and normalizing formula for the sexes. The ability to sustain relationships is still a psychiatric criterion of normality, despite the large instability of relationships in contemporary culture. Finally, Seminar XIX is also Lacan's continued exploration of the relationship between the One of the Real and of jouissance and the knowing associated with the Unconscious now conceived as something beyond the signifier and the Freudian unconscious. Lacan's Real unconscious, and its *savoir*, also has links with mystical forms of jouissance as Lacan himself has stated and Miller (2016, p. 182) has emphasized despite Lacan's earlier rejection of the ineffable and the existential/phenomenological focus on immediate experience. Despite the fact that Zen emphasizes 'ex-soteric' everydayness rather than esoteric otherworldliness, I have explored these themes (without the benefit of Seminar XIX) in a prior book on psychoanalysis and Zen Buddhism. Mysticism is typically otherworldly or is focused on the mysteries associated with God or a Deity. Zen instead is focused on the freedom of the heart and mind.

Chapter 9 explores the relationship between Lacanian psychoanalysis and the object relations school widely conceived. In contrast to France, Latin countries, and South America, Lacanians in the US have always been in interaction with the object relations school of psychoanalysis that grew out of the English-speaking world. The chapter is specifically focused on Winnicott given his similar interest on the individual as a true isolate. For Winniccott the latter is a product/fruit of the relationship with the mother while for Lacan it is a function of the Real and the lack of rapport between the sexes. In this regard, I must mention the efforts of Michael Eigen who for years held a Seminar in New York City on Bion, Winnicott, and Lacan.

Chapter 10 is my latest statement on the clinical practice of psychoanalysis. The latter is not just applied psychoanalysis, because the theory cannot be developed independently from the practice. Pure psychoanalysis could refer to interventions that are justified by theoretical criteria and not solely by practical rules. However, pure psychoanalysis should not be construed as only theoretical or academic since it also refers to the derivation of the theory from the unconscious signifying chain that is revealed in the actual singular practice of psychoanalysis. Finally, I would like to thank Magdalena Romanowicz for reading a prior unpublished version of this chapter, for pointing to the work of Hans Steiner, and the empirical literature on the clinical outcomes of psychoanalysis.

Chapter 11 was co-written with Dany Nobus and represents a response to an earlier paper of Dany's on Lacan and organizational theory in the light of my 27-year experience being a founding member and responsible person for the development of the first Lacanian School in the US under the leadership of Andre Patsalides who studied with

Lacan in Paris. At its foundation, the School had the support of the San Francisco Center for Psychoanalysis associated with the IPA, as well as of psychologists, who despite being practicing psychoanalysts, were denied official recognition by the IPA for not being MDs. Most notably Nathan Adler, a founding member of the School, was in analysis with Bernfeld, who migrated to San Francisco and had Freud's support but not of the American Psychoanalytic Association associated with the IPA. I took this opportunity to reflect on the experience of the School, and how it's development, problems, and promise, refer to the questions that Lacan articulated *a propos* of the School as a psychoanalytic organization.

Finally, I want to take this opportunity to thank the participants of my yearly Seminar at the Lacanian School for reading the chapters, giving me feedback, and the opportunity to sound off the ideas, and more clearly hear what I was trying to say in this book.

Berkeley, CA, USA Raul Moncayo

References

Lacan, J. (1972–1973). *On Feminine Sexuality. The Limits of Love and Knowledge, Book XX* (B. Fink, Trans.). New York and London: Norton.

Lacan, J. (1975–1976). *The Sinthome. The Seminar of Jacques Lacan, Book XXIII*, J. A. Miller (Ed.). Cambridge: Polity Press.

Contents

List of Figures

List of Tables

Introduction: Lacan's RSI and Freud's Two Theories of Mind with Three Dimensions

It is well known that Lacan's three registers/dimensions of experience (Real, Symbolic, and Imaginary or RSI) or psychical structure are knotted into a topological knot in such a way that if you untie one register the entire knot becomes untangled. But what about Freud's systems/instances? Do they also function in this way? None of the systems (in the topographical theory) or instances (in the structural theory) can exist without each other.

This book will couple basic concepts of Freudian and Lacanian theory and combine or stretch them in new ways and directions to illuminate not only the practice of analysis, applied to contemporary problems and conditions, but also its transmission in the psychoanalytic organization. While the book offers counterbalancing and divergent takes on Freud and Lacan, the work tracks a significant amount of psychoanalytic material, including ideas emerging from the object relations school (Chapter 9), and the relations of psychoanalysis with science and mathematics. The book underscores at every turn the traits that unite/separate psychoanalysis from other twentieth and twenty-first century schools of thought and practice.

At this point in the history of the field, there is no need for new introductions to Freudian or Lacanian theory since many have already been published and are readily available. This book will presuppose some basic concepts and will only define and expand on them in the context of providing new formulations for well-known concepts. Hopefully, the language and explanations will be clear enough to allow those with little or no prior knowledge of Freud or Lacan to find a rewarding way through the text.

In this book, I will follow Lacan's use of mathematical metaphors while not pretending or giving the impression that ordinary 'real' mathematics or arithmetical systems are primarily involved (Peano Axioms, or Principia Mathematica, for example). Mathematics as a field involves formulas that can be quantified and used within arithmetical systems. Lacan used the conceptual, logical, and non-empirical aspect of mathematics without the calculations/computations that make it an exact science. A psychoanalytic approach to mathematics is closer to Plato's conviction that other fields of knowledge had to be modelled after mathematics, than to the earlier Pythagorean use of mathematics to speculate about non-mathematical theory. Psychoanalysis does not need mathematics nor mathematics needs psychoanalysis, but psychoanalytic theory can be strengthened and made internally coherent by aspiring to make its theory consistent with conceptual mathematics and number theory.

Now does topological structure or the symbolic order constitute a system in the mathematical, or Gödelian, sense of the term? Does topological theory make Lacanian theory systematic as distinct from Lacanian theory being non-systematic? Non-systematic theory, as in Kierkegaard or Nietzsche, is not totalizing at the level of the Idea because there are intensities, affects, and jouissance that cannot be reduced to their ideational representatives. However, once these factors are considered and are built into the structure, then an open system can be incomplete yet consistent and systematic (see the definitions for these terms in Chapter 7).

Among other things, I intend to show how the structure of the Borromean knot can also be observed in the structure of the Mind/Psyche itself as conceived by Freud. Mind and psyche are not identical terms and thus already represent different dimensions/registers. For the Greeks psyche is the motivating aspect of mind while mind represents the aspect of the mind that maintains its equilibrium. While the psyche is dynamic and subject to frequent and high rates of change and disorder, the Mind is stable, orderly, and represents structures with a low rate of change.

These two dimensions of mind (drive and defense, psyche and mind) also re-appear in the contemporary study of the brain and the nervous system. The autonomic nervous system, that functions automatically as the name indicates, is subdivided into two systems: sympathetic and parasympathetic. The sympathetic nerve cells represent sexual arousal or psyche and mobilize energy for the 'Fight or Flight' reaction during stress, causing increased blood pressure, breathing rate, and blood flow to muscles. Conversely, the parasympathetic nerves have a defensive calming effect: they slow the heartbeat and breathing rate and promote digestion and elimination.

Both Mind and Psyche are found in Freud (in the form of desire and defenses), but what about Lacan, since Lacan is known to have rejected the notion of a well-integrated state of stable equilibrium? This perspective is relative given that in Seminar XI, when speaking of Freud's (1895) real ego (not the same as the reality ego), he defines it as a tendency to realize a balance of internal tensions. Lacan rejected the modern notion of ego autonomy derived from the humanistic individualism emerging from the Italian Renaissance. In the latter view, it was the ego's cultural function to introduce rational order and beauty into the chaos of the drives and nature instead of relying on traditional authority and the repression of the drive to do just that. For Freud, it was a matter of conscious control rather than unconscious and involuntary traditional repression.

For Lacan, language, law, numbers, and culture (the symbolic order) structures and 'orders' human subjectivity within society. What culture or the Other takes from the subject or the subject gives to the Other (*a*) generates a space for an entire system of social and linguistic exchange to take place at the level of the subject. This is the cultural significance of the symbolic phallic function of castration. The unconscious and the subject are heteronomous with respect to the ego. The subject is named by the signifier and represented by metaphor. But doesn't this violate the logic of modernity in favor of a traditional and even irrational form of authority?

The conflicts between the rational and modern demands of the ego for mutual respect, and the unilateral and hierarchical respect demanded by the traditional super ego, are negotiated in the social field of speech and language. With modernity, the focus of the moral agency is displaced to the individual subject and a sense of civic duty, and away from the external locus of control located in the social Other and the problems associated with guilt, shame, honor, social role, and status. In many ways, this process begun long time ago with Socrates and the invention of democracy in ancient Greece. Socrates in Greece, like the Buddha in India, and Confucius in China, around the same time, stressed personal responsibility rather than reliance on the gods or society.

However, once the focus shifts to the individual and his/her well-being (beauty and health values: hygiene, diet, esthetics, exercise), what appears to be moral autonomy from the societal Other turns into the question of autonomy or heteronomy with respect to the discourse of the Other of the unconscious. One of the things that have been discovered in the clinic of contemporary society, is that the less external control and censorship, particularly from parents (as representatives of the social order), the more tyrannical the internal super-ego may become. In addition, the external locus of control may shift from parents to peers who demand the very things that were forbidden by parents of a previous generation. The morality of postmodern peers demands jouissance as surplus satisfaction rather than privation and frustration.

Utilitarian morality is also demanded by the drive (i.e. the demand to enjoy embedded within the super ego of consumer capitalism as formulated by Lacan), technical reason (instruments that facilitate the satisfaction of needs and desires), and the internalization of culture despite the rejection of the same culture by more mature (rational and conscious) forms of the individual. For example, it is difficult, if not impossible, to differentiate unconscious censorship embedded within the very processes of representation and substitution, from the conscious moral dictates of ego representations.

Perhaps this is why Freud (1923), in the *The Ego and the Id* associated the unconscious of defense or repression with an unconscious ego: the nature of representation and the signifier (the Unconscious-Preconscious system abbreviated as Ucs.-Pcs.) is as rational as the organization of the ego can be. I say can be, because the ego also has unconscious aspects linked to the ego of narcissism and the drives at work within the ideal ego and the super-ego. When we speak of the moral agency of the ego, that appears to us autonomous with respect to the heteronomy associated with the social Other of society or Culture, such autonomy functions against the silent tacit background of the functioning of the Symbolic within language and kinship relations. The ego appears to be autonomous, and the subject heteronomous, but it all depends on reversible perspectives, and both are equally rational or consistent with reason.

The question of the super ego is something different and is rather associated with an irrational authority that appears arbitrary and solely based on force, violence, fear, and the whims of the Other, rather than rational virtue. The super ego uses aggressiveness to defend against aggressiveness, or fire to fight fire (i.e. only the state has the right to take life) and is therefore associated with the Id and the violence of nature and the primal father. Whether learning linked to the super ego represents the origin of rationality, or conversely whether the super ego forever remains separate from rational ethics, is something beyond the current purview of this book.

It is difficult to reconcile the reliance on a traditional symbolic order associated with symbolic castration and the phallic function, which invariably could be accused of being patriarchal (or linked to the primitive super ego), with Lacan's scalding critique of ego psychology and the hierarchical structure of the IPA that Lacan likened to the traditional structure of the Catholic Church. Lacan could conceive that the Symbolic order conditioned the fear of symbolic castration but rejected the hierarchical structure of the IPA.

Lacan also fantasized about an audience with the Pope, despite critiquing the hierarchical structure of the IPA and the Catholic Church. Despite his critique of the Catholic institution, Lacan considered the Catholic faith as the only "true religion", and he and his brother (as stated by his Jesuit priest brother during his funeral) believed that Lacan's 'doctrine' was consistent with the doctrine of the Catholic Church. In this respect, Lacan is not an innovator. This is a very modern condition whereby atheists who reject religion, are the very first to defend the traditional characteristics of religion as a culture. Although France is not primarily a Christian or Catholic country, like Spain and Latin America still are, they all share the fact that even if people identify as culturally Christian and are prepared to defend the Christian religion as the true religion, most declare themselves as atheists and hardly practice the religion that they are prepared to defend, nonetheless. The same is true in Israel, where secular Jews reject the orthodox variety of Judaism, but then very quickly rise to say that it is the only legitimate version of Judaism.

How to sort out this knot with contradictory strands? In his reliance on a pre-established traditional order, Lacan is a traditionalist. Although a symbolic order is not necessarily harmonious, it does represent an order as the name indicates. Lacan is also a traditionalist, nowadays, as far as his dogged allegiance to Freud's discovery of the Unconscious is concerned. However, Lacan's symbolic order or the Other is not a structure without lack, without fault lines, or a static structure not subject to change and transformation. The elements of the symbolic order have no positive existence because they are articulated by their differences or their emptiness or non-existence ('ex-sistence') as isolated individual elements. The relative identity of linguistic units/elements cannot have any influence on the empty and isolate nature of each unit, and therefore all they can do is depend on their relative identity and the combinations and interactions between them.

In addition, in the end and with the Real in sight, Lacan does attribute a dimension of un-determination to human experience linked to the structure of determination and over-determination found in Freud. Although Freud famously stated that the ego is not the master of his/her own house, Freud did give the ego a margin of autonomy and rational conscious control over the drives. Lacan instead locates un-determination within the register of the Real. Indetermination in mathematics refers to the x variable until numbers are computed by a formula or an arithmetical operation that produces an exact result or value for x.

This example would apply to automaton as only an apparent form of chance or undetermination that in fact is determined by the structure of number. The undetermined Real refers to *Tyché* as a true form of chance and randomness that can produce a new element or signifier within the structure, and a new structure, therefore.

The ego is included in the 'machinic' or cybernetic binary structure as a structure of facilitations and inhibitions within human experience. As I will show in Chapter 6, it is the structure that generates the possibility of an imaginary axis constitutive of the ego and the ideal ego. The undetermined subject of the Real is something different. The subject of the Real is found within the lack of the Other, or something missing and incomplete within the structure, that at the same time functions as the pivot for the evolution and involution of the structure. The storehouse structure of the Mind is made of causal series and results, subject and Other, things that work and don't work, evolve and devolve or decay. Chapter 8 develops a psychoanalytic theory of cognition and how it differs from cognitivism and the use of the digital computer as a guiding model. In contrast to a computer screen and a computational theory of mind, and although Lacan (1956) tried to use cybernetics to construct a model of the unconscious, a psychoanalytic theory of mind includes human aspects of experience and rationality that cannot be conveyed by the binary logic of a digital computer.

The subject of the Real must pass through the phallic function of castration which is the function that leaves something missing and un-symbolized within the structure (*l'a*). There (*là*) the subject finds itself as a form of jouissance and non-thinking, or non-knowing, that is also a different form of knowing, insight, and thinking. There is thinking and not thinking as refusing to think, and then there are various levels of thinking and reason: action/practice (practical reason), binary and dual thinking (formal reason), self-centred and objective thinking, nondual and dialectical thinking (dialectical reason), and non-thinking that includes thinking as well as vice versa (Nous).

So how is it possible that a Real subject can manifest a firm determination for something not necessarily included within an established symbolic order? How could scientific discoveries be possible otherwise? Thought and the signifier have been programmed according to rules of thought and computation and somehow a subject can think or not think something predicted by the *machinic* structure. This is the subject of jouissance and thought as a form of jouissance that leads subjects not only to symbolic knowledge and signification, but also to bliss and realization (as forms of the Third jouissance). So-long as they know how to practice, practitioners will find what they are seeking even if they don't seek. Lacan famously said (following Picasso), "I don't seek, I find." Here we do in fact find the subject and the unary trace as a vanishing point of equilibrium within the structure. Much like in Chaos theory (Prigogine, 1984), new orders are preceded by symptoms, contradictions, and the disequilibrium of the previous order.

The subject of the Real is a different form of agent, and master than the ego (S_0 rather than S_1). The suspended authority of the subject coincides in most respects with the figure of the analyst, who instead of appropriating the successes or failures of analysis and building an ego-identity out of them, becomes a subject or an object that vanishes or disappears from the internal structure of the analysand that underwent analysis. Rather than being like the S of the pure signifier that is incorporated into the signifying chain to realize the unconscious subject, the analyst is a pure signifier that is removed from the enduring and signifying structure of the analysand.

The mind as psyche represents everything that can be described as instinct, drive, desire, jouissance, the psychophysical complex, but as represented by images and linguistic signifiers. The object of the drive appears as images and forms but such images in humans are secretly determined by linguistic signifiers embedded within them. Mind itself is Symbolic or structural and is related to the Real as its vanishing point. On the other side (of the Borromean knot), the Symbolic is also related to the Imaginary in the form of ego structure and the ego's appropriation of the storehouse of the mind consisting of the seedbed of signs, images, signifiers, and numbers.

Mind represents the overall structure (including its inherent emptiness) as well as the seedbed and layers of inscription: icon/representation/significance (Imaginary, Symbolic, Real). This is Freud's metapsychological theory with the different systems of Mind functioning in space in the first theory (Ucs.Pcs.Cs.), and over time in the second theory of the personality (Id, Ego, Super ego), and the repetitions and reiterations between them. This book extends Freud's theory of representation into an understanding of the different levels of the signifying chain within Lacanian theory, and Freud's theory of the ego into the theory of the pure signifier of the subject in the Unconscious as a place of jouissance that adds the dimension of the senseless Real to the unconscious signifying chain.

The three categories in Freud's two theories of Mind and Lacan's Borromean Knot represent three dimensions that are tied and linked together and yet differentiated. The three systems in Freud (1915) are the Ucs.-Pcs., the Pcs.-Cs., and the Pcpt.-Cs., or the Unconscious-Preconscious, the Preconscious-Conscious, and the Perception-Consciousness systems. In the second theory, the three psychic instances, or aspects/moments/stages of the personality, are the Id, the Ego, and the Super Ego. Although these three are developmentally articulated, they are also included in each other in a way that is much more obvious than in the first metapsychological theory.

However, although the first theory is included in the second theory, the second theory is not included in the first. Perhaps this was Lacan's objection to the second theory. Following the imaginary aspect of a personality theory of the Mask or Semblance of a Mind, there are no obvious determining inscriptions or representations in the second theory other than the example of ego-representations.

In addition, the first theory has the metaphor of the magical writing pad, or a blank sheet of paper, or transparent membrane, or the empty mirror of the mind that corresponds to the Pcpt.-Cs. This instance is neither id (unless redefined as It) as a source of drives, nor ego, nor super-ego, in fact it may not even be a form of consciousness since consciousness is always consciousness of something. In this book, I will uphold this instance as a form of awareness linked to the evenly suspended, freely floating attention of the analyst that also represents a state of observation and broad mindfulness or psychical mindedness, as well as a form of jouissance. The Pcpt.-Cs. system is a luminous awareness beyond consciousness that has ties to the Real and to the push for emptiness as the unborn and undying Mind. This form of awareness is undetermined by the object of consciousness and because of this can clearly and objectively observe the determinations of consciousness and Mind in general.

The senses perceive objects in the external world according to the organ of sense involved and according to the Sense function at work in the various levels of psyche/mind, some conscious and some unconscious. The Sense function as the meaning function that regulates the significance of sense experience can also be attributed or appropriated by the subject, resulting in a symbolic identification. Nevertheless, the Sense function remains the Other that regulates the subject. Determination goes both ways but the Other precedes the subject.

A subject experiences sensation according to the sense modality, the material properties of the object, the physical waves and magnitudes, the numbers involved, and the words/sounds associated with them. In addition, sensations can be felt as pleasant, unpleasant, or neutral. It is the cognition and rationality at work in perception that distinguishes the various senses and their objects: this is a sound of…, this is the image of…, this is this body of…, that smells and tastes like….

The attribution of meaning to perception is something that comes from the subject and from the mental function of memory as it registers or inscribes, over time, and in layers, the personal and social history of the subject.

Registrations and inscriptions take place before there is a subject conscious of a determining object. It is the gradual and sudden manifestation of mental structure out of a storehouse of memories, that will lead to the development of various mental formations according to the Borromean knot: Imaginary fantasies and imaginations, the structure of physical/biological impressions and sensations, instincts and drives, unions and separations, desires and prohibitions or defenses, feelings of love and hate, logic/language and various levels of reason and knowledge. In this framework, the Real comprises the experience of the organism and the Real of the drive but as something more, as jouissance. At the core of instinctual and genetic determination there is something unconditioned or *a*causal as a push towards the emptiness of Being.

References

Freud, S. (1895). *A Project for a Scientific Psychology*. SE, 1, 283–397.
Freud, S. (1915). *The Unconscious*. SE, 14, 161–215.
Freud, S. (1923). *The Ego and the Id*. SE, 19, 3–66.
Prigogine, I. (1984). *Order Out of Chaos*. London: Shambala.

1

The Clear Screen, Perception, and the Nature of Inscription

In the Metapsychological papers where Freud (1915a) propounds his first theory of mind, he develops the topological/topographical distinction between three dimensions of Mind: Consciousness, the Preconscious, and the Unconscious which he respectively abbreviated as (1) Pcpt.-Cs.; (2) Pcs.-Cs.; and (3) Ucs. The problem of perception was central to Freud's first theory of mind. Freud conceived of the mind as having an unlimited receptive capacity for new perceptions and at the same time as having the capacity to lay down permanent memory traces of perceptions that become a seedbed or storehouse for new and repeated experience. The storehouse determines how the world is perceived, and at the same time is open to change thanks to the first system that remains open to new experience. He divided these two functions between two and three systems.

> Measured by this standard, devices to aid our memory seem particularly imperfect, since our mental apparatus accomplishes precisely what they cannot: it has an unlimited receptive capacity for new perceptions and nevertheless lays down permanent–even though not unalterable–memory-traces of them.

R. Moncayo, *Knowing, Not-Knowing, and Jouissance*, The Palgrave Lacan Series,
https://doi.org/10.1007/978-3-319-94003-8_1

> As long ago as in 1900 I gave expression in *The Interpretation of Dreams* to a suspicion that this unusual capacity was to be divided between two different systems (or organs of the mental apparatus). According to this view, we possess a system Pcpt.Cs., which receives perceptions but retains no permanent trace of them, so that it can react like a clean sheet to every new perception; while the permanent traces of the excitations which have been received are preserved in "mnemic systems" lying behind the perceptual system. (Freud, 1925)

Pcpt.-Cs. (Perception consciousness) is like a clear or empty transparent sheet/state that allows us to perceive the world in its pristine purity despite the fact that we have concepts and language to represent what we see and hear. Language and concepts (logic and numbers) are laid down in the first mnemic system known as the Pcs. or Pcs.Cs. (Preconscious conscious) since its contents are easily accessible to consciousness but are not in Pcpt.Cs. all the time.

To perceive there must be an empty layer (a clear sheet) that could receive impressions from the world without remaining saturated by the contents of the mind that already exist. There is an empty dimension of the mind that receives impressions but does not retain them and does not retain a representation even of itself, thus the metaphor of a transparent sheet that functions as a glass or membrane, more than a mirror. Writing, or memory functions on a layer or page beneath the covering sheet and it is where representations remain unless they are repressed, of course, in which case they disappear once again into the psyche in neurosis, and outside the psyche in psychoses.

What Freud calls a clean sheet is a metaphor for a psychical capacity, for a clear mind state or awareness that is the basis for listening and attention without interfering thoughts or memories or loud environmental stimuli. When we listen, we listen to the words and sounds, and the rest of our mind remains in the dark, in the background, as it were. We say this is the unconscious in a descriptive sense, all the words we know, or the memories and knowledge that we have that are capable of consciousness but that thanks to the clear state do not appear or interfere with conscious attention. The dynamic Freudian unconscious constitutes what within the Pcs.Ucs.

(Preconscious Unconscious) has been repressed and cannot be brought back to consciousness by an effort of will.

The clear sheet, celluloid, or awareness that represents Pcpt.Cs. is a protective shield against excitation that is also a definition that Freud gave of the ego. However, Freud's notion of the ego as a protective shield against stimuli or excitation highlights the defensive rather than the transparent function of the clear sheet. In the Metapsychology Freud first spoke of the perception-consciousness system (Pcpt.Cs.) and associated this clear sheet that does not retain impressions to consciousness and the state of being aware. This system or awareness as a clear state in the present moment without memory allows for the influx of new perceptions.

The Pcpt.Cs. and the Pcs.Cs. systems contain the awareness of new perceptions thanks to the clear transparent state of the mind, the acquisition of new impressions as a form of writing, and the protection provided by a shield against traumatic environmental stimuli (external world). The shield is also used against the disruption produced by perceptions and memories already laid down in the psyche that may threaten the clear sheet from within.

It remains unclear whether it is the transparent sheet that provides protection (the Pcpt.Cs. system), or the Pcs.Cs. system that tells us how and where to focus attention: "Attention!" A shield is not a celluloid sheet or a clear state although the latter can also inoculate us against external or internal perceptions by not retaining or holding on to them. In the Ego and the Id, Freud (1923) says that the Pcs.Cs. constitutes the nucleus of the ego. The ego is the protective shield (like the hardening surface of cheese) but secondary preconscious processes rule the ego more than the other way around as in the second formulation.

Freud also links the process of becoming aware or gaining consciousness to the awareness of feelings and thoughts that emerge within the subject. This corresponds to the Preconscious-Conscious (Pcs.Cs.) as distinguished from the Pcpt.Cs. system. Sometimes he also speaks of these as one and the same system. Memories or mnemic traces are contained both within the Pcs.Cs. and the unconscious (Ucs.). In addition, the Pcs. can also be considered Ucs. in a descriptive sense (the unrepressed Pcs.Ucs. system).

The defense involved in not retaining traces can be distinguished from the defense afforded by the Pcs.Cs. in the form of a stable receptacle of perceptions, memories, and modified thoughts that can also be used as a shield against the Ucs. and the surplus influx of stimuli and tension from without.

Lacan also uses the metaphor of a protective screen or more precisely the Symbolic order itself as a protective screen against the disruptive force of the Real as he initially conceived it. However, the Real is not the reality of the external world. The Real also refers to the Real of the drive and impulses emerging within the subject or subjectivity. Stimuli arise both from without and from within the subject. Finally, the Real is something empty of definition or that cannot be pinned down to a single definition.

In the case of the perceptual/conceptual system that is determined by the Pcs.Cs. more than the Pcp.Cs., it is difficult to distinguish between the external world and the external world as structured by language and perception. There is an aspect of the external world as *das Ding* or as things-in-themselves that remains outside the categories of perception. The "no-thing" is a form of non-perception or perception beyond the categories of perception. One could argue that this aspect of the Real also functions, as it were, as an empty movie screen on which we project our perceptions.

The screen of the Real in this sense facilitates the projective perception of a world and at the same time provides for a screening of the projection so that a constructive gap or hole can remain between perception as a construction of the social subject (or the Pcs.Ucs. system) and the Real of the things-in-themselves (the thing/no-thing). In the same way that the clear state of the transparent sheet does not hold on to impressions, the screen of the Real cannot be reduced to the Symbolic and Imaginary lenses through which it is seen or perceived. The screen of the Real represents the enigmatic dimension of truth and jouissance that never ceases from not being written.

Bristow (2017, p. 39), in his book on Joyce and Lacan, points out that Joyce said, when discussing his masterpiece Ulysses, that a transparent sheet separated his work from madness. The transparent sheet allows Joyce to recognize the madness and call it madness but not fall into it. In the example of James Joyce, since the Symbolic Pcs.Cs. protective shield, otherwise known as traditional character, did not function to protect Joyce against the internal or external worlds, Joyce had to rely on the transparent sheet or the Pcpt.Cs. and the screen of the Real against the madness of the world and his own personal demons/delusions. He could not trust Christian education or Irish society to come to his aid.

What passes through the transparent sheet is both a sense object/word and not an object/word since there is no code or cipher there in the same way that there are words that do not stick to the screen of the Real because the screen of the Real remains empty despite serving as a basis for projections. The word that is not a word, or the concept that is not a concept, or the number that is not a number, become hollowed out words that represent the hallowed screen of the Real or the clear state.

The Energetics/Dynamics of Thought and the Signifier

Now what is the difference between Pcs. and Ucs. representations, between structures in high or low rates of change? Are they the same representations that go through a transformation of their energetic state (economic or functional hypothesis) where the representations are experienced in a different light or is it rather that there are two different inscriptions that co-exist (topical hypothesis)? In addition, does the passage from the Pcs. system to the Ucs. system abolish the presence of the representation in the first system?

To address these questions, I must first begin with the current relevance of the concept of energy in Freud's work. Nowadays many see it as a dated physical concept of his time that reflected his attempt to conceive of psychoanalysis as a natural science. The concept of energy derived from thermodynamics is related to the psychodynamic and economic points of view within Freud's theory. Economics, for example, refers to the amounts (quanta/quota/sum) of energy in circulation in states of arousal, excitation, or thinking. Energy is not the same as feeling or sensation although feelings and sensations are not without levels or quantitative degrees of energetic intensity as subjectively experienced or measured by various physiological indicators. The concept of energetic intensity that cannot be reduced to feelings or sensations is like Lacan's concept of jouissance.

In physics, and to this day, energy is broadly divided into potential energy and kinetic energy. During Freud's time the steam engine was at the forefront of research in engineering, physics, and technology in general. Steam was an example of potential energy that Helmholtz called free energy, and kinetic energy represents the potential energy of steam put to work and transformed into the kinetic energy of the engine. Kinetic energy would be the equivalent of bound or quiescent energy. Free in this case meant potential energy that has not yet been applied or put to work. Free energy is put to work in practice and motion and paradoxically turns quiescent while it moves.

In contemporary neuroscience, energy is measured in terms of electricity running through the brain or chains of neurons. Electrical energy moves thanks to neurotransmitters that are released or not (open/close or on/off) into the nerve cell. They are released or not depending on oscillations and changes in the level of the electrical rest mass charge of the nerve cell that facilitate or inhibit the circulation of energy/electricity between neurons within the brain.

Potential energy is put into motion or changed into kinetic energy that runs and circulates along a nerve cell chain. Potential energy corresponds to the energy that is available in the rest state of the cell. These ideas are not necessarily inconsistent with the theory of energy in physics nor with the way that energy as electricity is discussed in neuroscience. However, in neuroscience and brain studies, and as far as I can tell, the concepts of energy in physics are not used the way that Helmholtz, Breuer (1893/1966) and Freud (1893/1966) used them to discuss the mind/psyche.

If we pair the two: the physical and biological/chemical forms of energy, the fluctuations in the levels of electrical charge, and the two types of energy described by Helmholtz and Freud what do we get? When a charge decreases, or increases, rises or falls, energy is not lost. The energy remains at the optimal level whether at rest in the cell or in the movement from cell to cell. Optimal level means stasis, the way that homeostasis, for example, works differently in the sympathetic and parasympathethic nervous systems.

In the sympathetic system stasis means arousal, and in the parasympathetic system stasis is quiescence or the bound state. The inhibition of an incoming impulse can happen by the non-release of a neurotransmitter into the synaptic gap or its re-absorption after it has been released. The facilitation of an impulse can take place by the release of a chemical element into the synaptic gap or the failure of the substance to be reabsorbed into the cell causing the impulse to lose its optimal level and degrade/decay into loose associations between ideas. Loose associations would represent entropy and decay.

Returning to base or rest level represents potential energy, and the energy is free, at rest, and available. And here we run into the paradox whether quiescence is when the energy is at rest or when the energy is applied and finds its stillness or optimal tension therein. I hope to have clarified this by indicating the differential function of the optimal level or homeostasis in the transmission/facilitation of electrical impulses and the inhibition of the same. Obviously, these questions will have to be answered by neuroscientists by determining the precise physiological mechanisms involved.

But in any case, free circulation requires that the cell return to base level once the impulse has been transmitted. In other words, conductivity must be inhibited once the firing of a neuron has been facilitated. If the chemical remains released or free in the sense of not inhibited or reabsorbed into the cell, then there is an overcharge that hinders the optimal charge of kinetic energy and thus the quiescence or stillness in movement and at base level is compromised.

The signifier, as Lacan defines it, working within signifying chains rather than chains of neurons, also has this inhibiting/facilitating function in terms of the symbolic elements of language and culture. In fact, since culture represents an equivalent of the natural environment for speaking beings, it may very well be, that the psychic symbolic environment of mind interacts with, if not determine, its equivalent terms at the level of cell functioning and structure. Skinner believed that humans could construct linguistic stimuli that would then acquire control over their behavior in the same way that natural external environmental stimuli could. The difference between Lacan and Skinner (1969) in this regard is that for Lacan, humans in each generation inherit language culturally or unconsciously (the Other) and do not acquire language by constructing linguistic stimuli out of their own conscious or behavioral agency only.

I underscore determination/conditioning or the cultural environment as a cause, because ordinarily in neuroscience the brain is assumed to be conditioning the mind. The cultural environment does not determine genetic sequence in DNA structure associated with the body or the organism. But modifications at the level of the nerve cell may be occurring because of the cultural environment that may, eventually, over a long period of time, affect gene sequencing. Such modifications within the cell, that may be as inborn as genes, are now part of the new biological discipline of epigenetics.

So, let's say that both the electrical synaptic impulse or action potential and the signifier that reveals/conceals desire, facilitates/inhibits, opens or closes the gates of action, uses or disuses certain laws and desires, both constitute regulatory principles of the body-mind Soma and the body-mind Mind. As earlier stated, we see here how the Symbolic system also functions as a gate keeper for a constant Name or Number that regulates and maintains a system's equilibrium/structure against a background of disequilibrium and change. There is dynamic change within a structure and then there is a different form of change when new elements lead to the destabilization of the previous structure and the emergence of a new one.

Potential and Kinetic Energy and Two Forms of Freedom and Binding

The two energies that Freud considers are free and bound. He borrowed the categories from Breuer (1893/1966), who borrowed them from Helmholtz, and to this day they remain foundational stones of the theory of energy in physics. Freud believed that free energy ruled or operated within the primary process in the Ucs., while bound or quiescent energy ruled or operated within the secondary process. Unlimited versus limited condensation and displacement distinguished the primary from the secondary process. Limited displacement and condensation allows for reversibility and memory. The primary process tries to eliminate tensions but in doing so creates more tensions and thus the mind has to learn to tolerate a low level of tension.

However, Freud inverted the two energies he received from Breuer. For Breuer in the unconscious the energy would not be free because of a fall in optimal tension. It remains bound to the thoughts and signifiers available in the Ucs. Conversely in the Pcs.Cs. system the energy would be free to circulate in optimal tension corresponding to a calm clear quality of symbolic thought.

The inhibition of an impulse at the level of a nerve cell, and the inhibition/concealment of desire by the signifier both produce an energy transformation that leaves the cell at a level of rest according to its mass. But the optimal tension at the level of rest or free energy makes the same ready for the facilitation of an impulse when the stimulus arrives.

The two meanings of potential and kinetic energy correspond to two different ways to understand the concepts of freedom and binding. Freedom can be freedom without restriction as a form of highly charged excitation over which the subject has little control (signaling the control that the object of the drive and desire has over the subject), or freedom can represent liberty within form and regulation. Lacan locates desire in the latter category. Desire and the Law intermingle. The first form of freedom represents how Lacan first came to understand jouissance. Conversely, bound or binding can represent stability and quiescence, or it can represent bondage and oppression. One meaning is positive and the other is negative.

Depression would be an example where defenses or homeostasis are oppressive. In depression, there is a lack of desire, of circulation, facilitation and conductivity. Within Lacanian psychoanalysis depression is understood, not only as the result of a loss but as a denial of the lack and this denial results in a lack of desire or conductivity of impulses whether within sensory or motor nerves. Depression as a symptom, that keeps the psychical system in a negative homeostasis or equilibrium, is the result of too much inhibition due to the sadistic super ego and a complicated and unresolved grief that results from a defense against loss or lack.

In addition, Freud considers these hypotheses as applied to the question of interpretation in analytic practice. When an interpretation makes a content of mind conscious, Freud assumes that it does not eliminate the unconscious effects of the same representations. But is there a change in the Ucs. inscription because of the second inscription in the Pcs. system that now makes the Ucs. representation capable of consciousness?

Using Lacan's graph of desire that contains two signifying chains crossing the vector of desire to constitute desire, we observe the upper unconscious signifying chain (Ucs.) running horizontally left to right parallel to the lower chain of defensive ego discourse or the Pcs.Cs manifest narrative (Fig. 1.1).

We see in the example of the graph of desire why the two horizontal chains would remain two rather than one being converted into the other. There is a change in inscription and structure between the two chains. From the Other scene that could be obscene, but not necessarily, to the socially acceptable or "coded" narrative. The ego is involved in the latter, or the chain of discourse, while the upper signifying chain

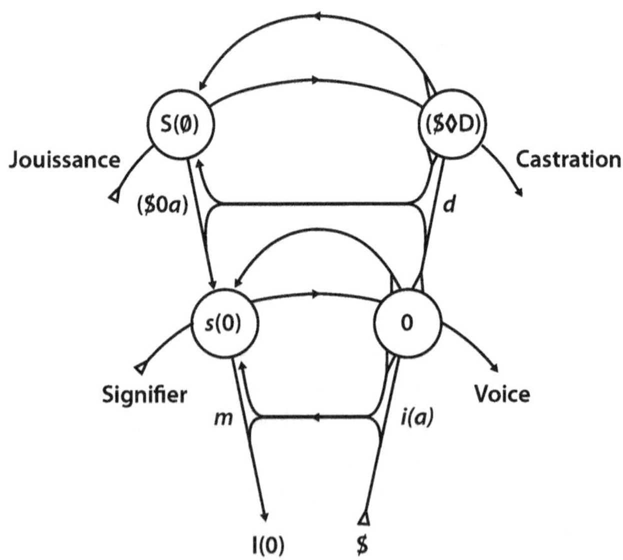

Fig. 1.1 Complete graph of desire. Romanowicz and Moncayo (2015)

contains the pure Signifier (S) as a representation of the subject in the place of jouissance.

This is the difference in the representation or the inscription/writing that Freud was asking about. Now does analysis convert one into the other, or are both changed by the interaction, yet in the end remain two separate chains? The latter seems the most likely scenario. If the Ucs. signifying chain would be converted into the manifest social narrative, then the Ucs., as the creative force, would be lost in translation to the ego. Would this be so bad if the Ucs. represents the id or the primitive cauldron of impulses that need to be transformed into a civilized state?

Well the problem is that this is a very limited view of the Ucs. The Ucs. works within language rather than simply representing a kind of primitive biological energy reservoir. Nevertheless, the *Je* of the unconscious differs from the I of the ego within a narrative or story. The Subject/Signifier (S) in the Ucs. gives access to a dimension of lack and desire that interacts with the biological demands of the drive and with the desire of the Other and the Other as such, including its inconsistencies and lack. The function of the signifier in the Ucs, is a Lacanian concept because for Freud unconscious representations solely consisted of thing representations by which he meant images that represent a part or aspect of a reality object.

Now what about the change in energy investment or cathexes of the drives as they relate to the two representations, inscriptions, and the two forms of energy? The two inscriptions would have to belong to the principle by which the organism presents demands/stimulus to the mind (psychical apparatus as Freud called it). The mind responds by producing thoughts, images, representations, and linguistic signifiers. From this point of view both inscriptions would work with kinetic energy in circulation or motion. Free energy would remain outside representation like the Real of jouissance in Lacan's work.

Another alternative hypothesis that Freud considers is the passage of a representation from one system to another mediated by the intervention of consciousness. In this case, there is both a change of energetic state and a double inscription. I think that what Freud might have in mind here is the hypothesis of primary repression at the origin of the psychical system within an ontogenetic and individual line of development. The moment we are looking for is the moment of the appearance of the first representation with less consideration to the fact that it may be inborn or not.

A presentation could be of the internal or external worlds, but consciousness appears to be directed by the evolutionary necessity to relate to an external environment, whether natural or cultural. Freud emphasizes the Pcpt.Cs. system as the first system. A mother is an example of the first natural and cultural environment/object. The desire of and for the mother would apply to both. The first representation of the object of the drive begins to develop around the Pcpt.Cs experience of satisfaction at the breast and its consequent loss when the breast is absent.

The separation from the breast generates the fantasy of the object (of desire) and its loss and the consequent symbolization of the object of desire and the cause of its disappearance. The fantasy of the object and its lack is an example of repressed Ucs. inscriptions, while the symbolization of both conforms the Ucs.Pcs. system. The unconscious in this case represents the descriptive rather than the repressed dynamic unconscious (Ucs. proper). From the point of view of Lacan's paternal metaphor $(\frac{\textit{Name of Father}}{\textit{Mother's Desire}})$, the Ucs.Pcs. system inscribes the Name of the Father and its branches, and the Ucs. proper inscribes the first signifiers of desire. In the Lacanian Borromean knot, the unconscious could not only be an imaginary phenomenon consisting of image-representations. The latter would be the Freudian perspective since Freud assigned language to the secondary Pcs.Cs. system, and images to the primary process in the Ucs.

In Lacan the signifier also functions in the unconscious through the subject of the Ucs. In the Ucs. the S is more of an instance of desire in time than a spatial intrasubjective structure or agency like the ego. Signification and significance is still operative in the Unconscious in the form of *lalangue*, the equivocal or antithetical use of a single signifier, the operations of metaphor and metonymy, and the ways that the Law and separation are represented.

These modes are observable in dreams and in speech. In addition, the formulation regarding the Subject/signifier in the Ucs., also explains the enigmatic knowing that is conveyed and contained in dreams. Sometimes a fresh thought/signifier from the ancient/present

Ucs. is the best thought in the direction of the Real instead of a regurgitated secondary elaboration according to secondary process thinking. Homeostasis or optimal quiescence is realized in a state of primary arousal instead of an unrealized threshold potential due to a state of rest or inhibition. When optimal quiescence is not achieved in a state of rest, then it may be realized in an instance of optimal tension in the Ucs.

On the other hand, often there are times when optimal arousal is not achieved in the Ucs. and the result is the usual association of the Ucs. with the archaic and primitive mentality where the subject may end up saying: "What was I thinking, or I wasn't thinking when I was amid an impulsive state of arousal and agitation". Thinking in this case refers to the realistic formal logical thinking of the ego and the secondary process where quiescence and binding is achieved. Thus, a quiescent energy or state is not a permanent feature of the secondary process nor is free energy a permanent state of the primary process. Sometimes optimal tension is realized in the Ucs. and not in the Pcs., and sometimes, or often, optimal tension is realized in the Pcs-Cs.

Free energy also means that energy is free to be converted into kinetic excitation by the switch that regulates the swinging door between inward and outward currents, internal and external environments at the cell level or between subjective and objective environments or the subjectively perceived environment or Umwelt as von Uexküll described it (von Uexküll, 1987). Umwelt or a bubble or membrane may be a better term to describe the Pcpt.Cs. system than the conventional notion of an ego. The bubble or umwelt in which the organism lives is not solipsistic because it represents the subjectively perceived external world. The umwelt bubble is a three-dimensional unconscious image, while the specular image or body image is only two dimensional. A current surprising observation consistent with the Umwelt as a three-dimensional body image, is the study of soldiers or people who have lost limbs and yet continue to have sensations in the limbs that are no longer there. This has been explained as an unconscious or mental body image that interacts with the physiological organism and that is still there in its entirety despite the fact that some limbs of the physical body have been lost. The sensations are experienced in the mental Umwelt body that mediates the relation to the external environment.

If free energy does not rise to the threshold level, then the energy is not free to accept an incoming stimulus and what should be converted into kinetic energy is not. The optimal base level of free energy would allow for the absence of inscription that is the physiological/energetic correlate of the Pcpt.Cs. system that we mentioned above: the capacity of the Mind to remain free of inscriptions to process new perceptions. When free energy is in a degraded non-optimal state then free energy would not allow or would not cease in the capacity to not register inscriptions representing thereby, in this case, the pathological aspect of defenses.

Moreover, can the energies transform from one system to another, or do structural energies remain the same and it is the representation that is detached from one energy and reinvested with another? We saw that kinetic energy can be optimal or not optimal in either system of inscription. Inscriptions in the Ucs. system will function differently depending on whether the level of kinetic energy is optimal or not. The same is true for the inscriptions in the Ucs.Pcs. system, the inscriptions will function differently depending on whether kinetic energy is at the optimal level or not.

The opposite hypothesis would be that it is the type of representation that determines the type of energy and feelings existing in both systems. Are feelings and actions the result of the quality of the representational element? And how to differentiate this from the case where representations vary by the nature of the energy linked to them? It seems representations vary by the signifier at play and the quality of energy at work in the system. The signifier associated with the representation of the object can vary and so can the type of level associated with kinetic energy.

Quiescence or optimal tension associated with kinetic energy in the Ucs. or Pcs. systems would lead to benevolent or pleasant forms of excitation, while the failure to achieve the optimal level in both systems would be expressed in the form of unpleasant feelings. In the Ucs., representations and signifiers of desire are accepted and facilitated and in the Pcs. they are not. If the facilitation or the inhibition is not optimal, in such a way that facilitation is followed by inhibition and inhibition is followed by facilitation, then the excess facilitation and the excess inhibition will be experienced as unpleasant.

An unpleasant feeling is a sign that facilitation did not stop, and that the cessation of the stimulus is not followed by facilitation. Now what does this have to do with the quality of the representation?

The pleasant/unpleasant quality of the signifier in the Ucs is determined by the facilitation of desire but for this facilitation to remain optimal it must alternate between movement/facilitation and stillness/inhibition. Inhibition functions in the Ucs. in the same way that facilitation functions in the Pcs. Although the Ucs. typically involves cultural representations of desire, and the Pcs. involves cultural representations of the Law, there is law or inhibition within desire and facilitation or desire within the Pcs. system. We don't desire without the Law, and the Law is also another form of desire.

The question that follows is whether the energetic and physiological mechanisms associated with the type of energies involved can be considered interpretants or signifieds within a symbolic system (as Peirce believed) or whether they lie outside the signifying symbolic system. The answer is that the energies and jouissance remain outside the signifying system, yet the energies can suffer predictable transformations in relation to key signifiers functioning with the Symbolic. This is a case where the signified would be in the Real of the body.

Feelings, however, are not outside the representational system since they are also a response to external cultural others and their speech. Feelings are mediated by the representational system of the subject and the symbolic battery of signifiers. In addition, a subject can mistake the interpretation or meaning of the affect. The conscious ego can attribute a meaning to the speech of the Other and experience a feeling or impact as an effect, but the interpretation does not come from the affect but from repressed signifiers that are signifiers nonetheless. The energetic or jouissance aspect of the affect is in the Real but the affect is an interpretant or a signifying element. The signifiers in the other's speech mediated by unconscious signifieds of the subject provide an interpretation for the affect.

For Lacan the Name of the Father (NoF) as a signifying/representational element produces the binding associated with the link between representations. In the final analysis, the question whether the binding comes from the representation or from the type of energy is circular because in the formula for the discourse of the analyst, the analyst appears as the *objet a* in the Real ($\frac{a}{S_2}$) and in the numerator place of the agent. The NoF and knowing or *savoir* as the denominator (S_2) are in the place of truth. The *objet a* in the Real represents infinite Life that supports the binding/linking energy of the signifier of the NoF as well as vice versa. In the paternal metaphor ($\frac{S_2}{S_1}$) the *a* in the discourse of the analyst is presented as S_1 and the places are inverted so that the NoF appears as signifier and the desire of the mother as signified. The S_1 for the desire of the mother appears as either the object of the mother's desire as signified (the imaginary phallus) or as pure desire that would be the same as *objet a*.

I can conclude that the NoF is at the junction of two forms of Infinity, one associated to the generation of signifiers for the desire of the mother and the *objet a* (cause of the mother's desire) according to Lacan's symbolic equation for the relationship between the *objet a* and the phallus: *a*/-phi. The *a* attempts to close the gap of the minus phi. The fractioning of the *objet a* and its displacement into new signifiers can be represented numerically by irrational numbers on the x axis, the decimals of which continue to infinity.

But what stops this form of infinity is the function of the Name and the process of nomination. Phi is a name regardless of the number of decimals that defines it, and the same could be said of Pi. A Name places a boundary but thinking of the Name as a finite boundary (sometimes known as 'finitism') has the limitation of ignoring the function of the NoF and the possibility of the Name opening the door to a different form of infinity that is ubiquitous or found everywhere. The notion of the NoF as a finite boundary corresponds to the notion of the NoF or the symbolic order as a static order not subject to change. The NoF as opening the door to the Real as a ubiquitous infinity is precisely the place of change and permutation for the structure of the Symbolic order. In this case, the Symbolic order changes not only in extension but also in structure.

The first form of infinity follows from the non-existence of the symbolic phallus. Because the symbolic phallus is the signifier of a lack or the lack of a signifier (for the phallus), then this leads to a continuous displacement and fractioning of the *objet a* and the imaginary phallus (both of which stand for one of the two golden numbers: phi, and—phi). When the capital Phi is applied as a Name, then its number stops or subtracts the phi (1.618-0.618 = 1). The 1 that exists within the infinity of Real and irrational numbers is a different number in the complex plane because it circles into the axis of imaginary numbers. This point will be further explained in chapter VII. The second form of infinity can be found in the timelessness of the Unconscious where past present futures exist at the same time. We can look at time from the perspective of a continuous sequence or travel time, but we can also perceive it as a sequence of discontinuous now's that are all the same now however many times it can be instantiated or iterated. In his thought experiment of travelling on a ray of light, Einstein also found that at *c* or the speed of light, time stands still.

References

Bristow, D. (2017). *Joyce and Lacan: Reading, Writing, and Psychoanalysis*. London: Routledge.

Freud, S. (1915a). *The Unconscious*. SE, 14, 161–215.

Freud, S. (1915b). *Repression*. SE, 14, 143–158.

Freud, S. (1923). *The Ego and the Id*. SE, 19, 3–66.

Freud, S. (1925). *A Note Upon the "Mystic Writing-Pad"*. SE, 19, 227–232.

Freud, S., & Breuer, J. (1893 [1966]). *Studies on Hysteria*. New York: Avon Books.

Romanowicz, M., & Moncayo, R. (2015). Going Beyond Castration in the Graph of Desire. *The Letter (The Irish Journal for Lacanian Psychoanalysis)*, *58*(Spring), 31–58.

Skinner, B. F. (1969). *Contingencies of Reinforcement: A Theoretical Analysis* (p. 283). New York: Appleton-Century-Crofts.

von Uexküll, T. (1987). The Sign Theory of Jakob von Uexküll. In Krampen, et al. (Ed.), *Classics of Semiotics* (pp. 147–179). New York: Plenum.

2

Instinct and Drive in Darwin and Freud, Contemporary Psychoanalysis and Biology

This chapter revisits the relationship between Darwin (1859) and Freud given that nowadays Darwinian principles play a greater in biology than ever before. Darwin's theory of natural selection lacked an adequate account of inheritance and thus once genetic mechanisms were identified (following Mandel's work), evolutionary genetics became a central part of biology. Studies of natural selection that use DNA sequence data are answering questions first asked by Darwin.

However, the dangers of the synthesis between Darwinian ideas and genetics is the temptation to reduce the social sciences and the humanities to biological and physical phenomena. When this reduction is enacted, very controversial and primitive views emerge about gender, sex, race, and culture, that conflict with the more properly human notions of culture found within the social sciences, the humanities, and psychoanalysis. This chapter argues that it is precisely psychoanalysis that needs to be used by the social sciences and the humanities to understand culture in symbolic terms that cannot be reduced to biology and yet can interact with the biological determinants of instinct and inheritance in human beings.

R. Moncayo, *Knowing, Not-Knowing, and Jouissance*, The Palgrave Lacan Series,
https://doi.org/10.1007/978-3-319-94003-8_2

In his Metapsychological papers, Freud (1915) proposed that protofantasies or primal fantasies, such as intrauterine life, seduction, the primal scene, and castration, are innate and the product of experience that was laid down during the cultural evolution of the species once the specific biological species had manifested. This is not the place to elaborate and explain the various fantasies but enough is to say that Freud's conception of primal fantasies covers both primal scenes as environmental events as well as psychical fantasies that structure how environmental events are perceived and constructed. Biological and physiological evolution leading up to the human form concerns DNA and the structure of genes. An acquired characteristic may be innate and passed on through sexual reproduction but without being part of the gene structure.

Freud's (1921) theory of the primal horde, that he developed under the influence of Darwin's ideas, represents another example of something acquired that can be unconsciously and innately passed down through the generations without being part of the gene structure.

> In 1912 I took up a conjecture of Darwin's to the effect that the primitive form of human society was that of a horde ruled over despotically by a powerful male. I attempted to show that the fortunes of this horde have left indestructible traces upon the history of human descent; and, especially, that the development of totemism, which comprises in itself the beginnings of religion, morality, and social organisation, is connected with the killing of the chief by violence and the transformation of the paternal horde into a community of brothers. To be sure, this is only a hypothesis, like so many others with which archeologists endeavour to lighten the darkness of prehistoric times—a 'Just-So Story', as it was amusingly called by a not unkind critic (Kroeger); but I think it is creditable to such a hypothesis if it proves able to bring coherence and understanding into more and more new regions.
>
> Human groups exhibit once again the familiar picture of an individual of superior strength among a troop of similar companions, a picture which is also contained in our idea of the primal horde. The psychology of such a group, as we know it from the descriptions to which we have so often referred—the dwindling of the conscious individual personality, the focussing

> of thoughts and feelings into a common direction, the predominance of the emotions and of the unconscious mental life, the tendency to the immediate carrying out of intentions as they emerge—all this corresponds to a state of regression to a primitive mental activity, of just such a sort as we should be inclined to ascribe to the primal horde. (Freud, 1921, p. 54)

These ideas are inferred but are also based on observations of patient's speech in analysis that are not based on introspection, because they require the Other to recognize them. Otherwise they remain obscure and irrational aspects of human experience that remain unexplained. The observations are singular in that the individual cannot recognize them through introspection alone, and although they appear in dreams the individual needs the analytic situation to make them conscious. The same material can be observed in many individuals although the sample size of cases in psychoanalysis may not be large enough to produce significant statistical results. In addition, the phenomena observed in individuals can also be observed in the patterns of group life.

> In Chapter VII of the *Origin of Species*, Darwin proposed that instincts were behavioral adaptations that had evolved by natural selection and sexual selection. …In his later book, On the Expression of Emotions in Men and animals, Darwin explained the roles that emotions play in the biology of animals and extended those explanations to humans. He argued that emotions are essentially biological processes analogous to other physiological adaptations, and that the methods by which they can be studied are similar to those by which any other inherited trait can be scientifically analyzed. (MacNeill, 2009, http://evolpsychology.blogspot.com/2009/03/summary-in-chapter-vii-of-origin-of.html)

The problem with extending explanations for animal dispositions to humans is that the symbolic or psychical/mental dimension of dispositions may be lost. Mind and drive in human beings must be understood in relationship not only to natural but also cultural and symbolic environments.

The concept of mind contains a reference to the hidden structure of physical impressions, sensations, impulses or drives, feelings or affects than can be pleasant, unpleasant, or neutral.

How do feelings or affect, for example, contain both physiological dispositions/mechanisms, affect as a representative of bodily or organic processes, and affect as determined by the cultural environment and the relationship to others mediated by language.

Feelings are not only the effects that the words and actions of others have on the subject, but also how the words and actions of others interact with the impulses, desires and drives of the subject as their signified or meaning. In other words, what the words of the Other mean to the subject not only has to do with the saying and the said of the enunciation of the other but also with the desires and drives of the subject that act as interpretants or signified for the words of the Other.

Out of this interaction feelings/sensations may become pleasant, unpleasant or neutral. Emotions, in turn, can be defined as the reactive actions towards the other based not only on the words and actions of others but also on the desires and fears, impulses and drives of the subject.

Darwin initially avoided defining instincts directly and instead spoke of them as behaviours. But behaviour for behaviourists is usually a learned or acquired response to the environment while instinct includes behaviours that are inborn or innately determined. Instincts are not acquired or learned via experience. Instincts are inborn dispositions.

> Individuals who have never learned how to perform them, nor experienced the same set of stimuli before in their lives can perform instincts. (Eliciting behaviours from animals that have been raised in isolation proved this.) Finally,…instinctive behaviours do not seem to require judgment or reason on the part of the individuals performing them… By implication, this means that instincts are essentially unconscious; that is, they are not the result of conscious deliberation or intentions. (idem)

Darwin also distinguished between instincts and habits. Habits are acquired by constant repetition, a repetition that can become an unconscious compulsion. However, Darwin also believed that some habits could be inherited. In this respect, evolution could at least partly proceed by the inheritance of acquired characteristics, something that Lamarck (1809) had argued prior to Darwin with his theory of inheritance of characteristics acquired through effort and will.

However, Weismann (1889-whom Freud [1920] cites) showed that anatomical characteristics are genetic rather than acquired. Weismann conducted the experiment of repeatedly removing the tails of mice and reported that no consequent mice were born without a tail or even with a shorter tail.

On the other hand, as Darwin believed, and the new field of epigenetics has discovered, mental or cultural traits or circumstances in life that are learned or acquired through repeated habit can also cause genes to be silenced or expressed over time. Cultural traits in humans, such as psychical sexual difference, and social gender roles, can turn on or off genetically determined differences between the sexes.

In addition, there have been indications that some epigenetic changes can be inherited. Learned behaviour may be passed on through several generations without the requirement for a change in genes at all. Given enough time, chance mutation may enable the genes to catch up with and consolidate phenotypic change. This new point of view that gives support to both Darwin's and Lamarck's theories is what is now known as the field of epigenetics.

Darwin believed that some emotional expressions are the result of repeated habit that eventually became hereditary. Darwin used cultural objects such as the camera and the photograph to study the facial expression of human emotion. The camera stands for observation, and how emotions themselves are produced in relationship to the other, but where the Other is a cultural structure and not necessarily another member of the same species.

For Darwin, natural and sexual selection were both equal mechanisms for evolutionary change (Rose & Rose, 2010). Sexual selection is supposed to explain psychological gender differences between women and men. Men were hunters, but women were food-gatherers, for example. Feminist anthropologists have challenged this assumption as a norm within the animal kingdom at least in certain species. Zihlman (2012) has noted the hunting and tool using skills of female primates.

Although sexual selection appears to be just as inborn as natural selection, the examples that Darwin uses in animals and humans are far from clear in terms of evaluating the relative influence of nature and cultural environment on sexual reproduction.

Not only do genes adapt to their environment but also environment adapts to genes. By environment what is meant here is not only the natural environment but also, and more importantly for speaking beings, the social and cultural environment mediated by language.

Paradoxically, the highest point of the tree of life is not the human organism but the cultural organization of *Homo sapiens*. Nonetheless, as Geertz (1973) pointed out, it is more likely that culture influenced human evolution, rather than simply thinking that culture was invented by humans who had already acquired the essential ingredients of modern human anatomy. Tool manufacture would be an example of this.

But what do I mean by culture in this book? Obviously on the manifest or phenomenological anthropological level and common sense, culture is associated with thinking, feelings, beliefs, rituals (secular or sacred), ideals, the normative regulation of human activity, art, fashion, culinary culture, etc. Within psychoanalysis beliefs fall under the rubric of the ego ideal structured by identification with cultural ideals.

Dawkins (1976) developed the concept of a replicator that would be more general than the gene and could also be used to explain the replication of cultural actions and activities that are passed on from one generation to the next by non-genetic means. The replicator is identical to the concept of imitation and Dawkins coins the term *meme* to place it on a parallel and structural level to the concept of gene.

> "We need a name for the new replicator, a noun that conveys the idea of a unit of cultural transmission, or a unit of *imitation*. 'Mimeme' comes from a suitable Greek root, but I want a monosyllable that sounds a bit like 'gene'. I hope my classicist friends will forgive me if I abbreviate mimeme to *meme*.... Examples of memes are tunes, ideas, catch-phrases, clothes fashions, ways of making pots or of building arches. Just as genes propagate themselves in the gene pool by leaping from body to body via sperms or eggs, so memes propagate themselves in the meme pool by leaping from brain to brain via a process which, in the broad sense, can be called imitation." (Dawkins, 1976, p. 192)

The psychoanalytic term would be identification rather than imitation. Identification is more than imitation, since for Lacanian theory, imitation would be an imaginary form of identification. In imitation there is a sense of copying the Other, and sometimes pretending to be the person imitated. Imitation can lead to the impostor syndrome. Identification instead implies the development of a separate identity. As Freud (1917) says in *Mourning and Melancholy*, identification is how the subject comes to separate from its objects. Through memory the ego appropriates the contents of the Other (a battery of signifiers) and misrecognizes the Other as self.

But the more operative and structural notion of culture in psychoanalysis is more consistent with structural anthropology (Levy-Strauss, 1949) that conceives the cultural order as organizing symbolic exchanges involving privileges and responsibilities, laws and entitlements, power and obligations, various prohibitions and the right of use of objects of enjoyment. As I showed in Chapter 1, this structure of facilitations and inhibitions, is shared by the brain, mind, and culture. Such structure is operative in language, in kinship relations, marriage, gifting, and economic exchanges. Culture is a system of meanings and symbols, a veritable signifying structure, but is also composed of psychical structures that determine and orient human activity. An intersection between signifying and psychical structures provides a good description of the psychoanalytical field.

In general, this book follows a methodological distinction between the Imaginary, the Symbolic, and the Real. The Imaginary is *how* the structure or the elements (*what*) of the structure appear in a phenomenon. The structure of interaction between facilitations and inhibitions, appear as ideas and values that are transmitted between the generations. The structure determines the beliefs although the structure appears absent from the conscious relationship to social beliefs. From the point of view of conscious experience and the social narrative about beliefs, the structure appears absent or non-existent although its apparent non-existence does not stop its Real structure ('ex-sisting' or non-existing) from effectively generating how the structure appears and disappears.

An example of the cultural environment, which serves as a poor and imaginary example of cultural development, is the racial hierarchy that existed in the British Empire between the so-called Savages of South America and the so-called higher European civilization. Darwin also thought that whites would out-evolve blacks.

In Darwinian theory, sexual selection explains the differences between the sexes within a single species. But here difference has all the ugly consequences that women often reject as representing the claimed superiority of the male over the female. Males compete and fight over females. Females then choose the strongest, smartest, or most beautiful male. This serves to ensure the reproduction and selection of male characteristics that females find most attractive. Males then evolve stronger and more powerful characteristics that seem to reify a biological basis for the subordination of women under powerful males. The same arguments have been made regarding the master-slave difference between whites and blacks or indigenous natives.

From a Darwinian and biological point of view there is no problem in saying that human males prefer younger women with low waist-hip ratios and females prefer older, richer, and more powerful males. This is the pure biological explanation except for the fact that it is loaded with cultural implications as to what instinct represents at the cultural level. Therefore, Freud posed the question of civilization, and civilization and its discontents, in relationship to the drive and how the drive itself may be affected by what Lacan called the Symbolic order.

When the structural question of the difference between the sexes translates into cultural or societal manifestation it acquires quite a different meaning. For example, if you said, following Darwin and biology, that younger females prefer sex and reproduction with older males, nowadays this is something that the culture rejects as a manifestation of the domination of one gender over another (something that naturally happens in the animal species). Here feminists are split between those who argue that patriarchy is a human construction to favour the interests of men and is not a phenomenon found widely across the animal realm, to those who agree and accept that male domination is found in nature but that as human beings we have to rise above and beyond it. I tend to agree with the second argument.

In Darwinian biology, differences in natural and sexual selection are construed as simply the struggle for the violent survival of the fittest or the stronger and dominant white males over female and 'racially inferior' counterparts. Even products of human culture, such as art, religion, and ethics, are conceived as manifestations of genes, natural selection, and neural processes in the brain.

This is precisely the point where culture and cultural ideals intervene. In humans, power must be eventually legitimized by ideals of equality and justice. Strength and power is no longer sheer force, cruelty, and domination, but also forms of rationality that cannot be reduced to instrumental cognitive interests. In the social contract as conceived by Hobbes (1668) and Freud, the avowal and acceptance of cultural ideals or ruling ideas has the same function of guaranteeing the survival of the species as a mechanism taking place in the relations between a group or society and its leader.

For Hobbes, the individual relinquished homicidal wishes and actions towards leaders and authorities, and adopted the precepts of civilization, in exchange for receiving the protection of the leader and the state. In Freud (1913) the primal horde of brothers restored the murdered father to the status of a totem and a set of beliefs, partly out of guilt, and partly to prevent the cycle from repeating all over again between new leaders and followers.

Here we observe a good example of how cultural environment affects the expression of natural dispositions and instincts. Culture seems to have an epigenetic characteristic in the sense of how genes can evolve or at least not evolve but interact with molecular cell mechanisms that modulate/mediate the manifestations and repercussions of mental or cultural traits that can be passed on and inherited. Phenotypal expression of the genes constitute a kind of second nature that emerges as an interaction between nature and cultural environment.

Freud believed that what he called the super ego as a cultural acquisition could be inherited. The super ego is the inner conscience, the seat of primitive morality, and the internal representative of culture within the psyche/brain of the individual. Such and like hypotheses are often used and abused by nations who see themselves as born with a higher potential for discipline and development. One can think of the Jews who believed themselves to be born with a superior soul; the Japanese who believe they come directly from the sun; the Chinese and the Japanese for centuries considered the rest of the world as barbarian and uncivilized; the Germans, whom Hegel thought embody the purest expression of human reason in their national spirit; and the English, who during the British empire also saw themselves as the pinnacle of culture and civilization. Finally, North Americans with their doctrines of manifest destiny and American exceptionalism represent another version of the same phenomenon.

Obviously, the problem with these views is that they can very easily and directly lead to toxic notions of racial superiority that underestimate the plasticity of human nature and the possibility and ideal that various races and cultures could eventually, and under the right genetic and environmental conditions, attain the ideals of human culture and civilization. In any case, some of the attainments of culture (kindness and equality, for example), can also be found in animals and non-educated human beings, however rare, random, or contextual these observations may be.

Now can we say that fairness and kindness are acquired cultural characteristics of civilized (repressed) society or to the contrary argue that these are traits that are also found in animals and therefore are innate, instinctual, or natural? Freud believed the former although there are biologists and ethologists who believe that kindness has survival value for the group and therefore also for the individual. Thus, kindness or positive emotion may also be an instinctual and involuntary disposition. Kindness and cruelty can be equally observed in animals.

For Freud, maternal tenderness or kindness was a drive and a primary form of object relation, although he initially conceived it as the expression of a self-preservation ego drive. If kindness is a primary form of object libido even before there is an object, or a subject for that matter, how could it be an ego drive other than the fact of being different from sexual drives?

If kindness is observed in animals and apes, then kindness is an instinctual element, a primary material that culture and the environment interact with. Under Freud's second theory of drives, where the ego drives disappear, and the ego is subsumed under the Life or Death drives, it is clearer to see maternal tenderness as a manifestation of the Life drive. Although sexuality is Eros, Life as Eros is more than sexuality since sexuality also works under the death drive. And although sexuality is part of the death drive (the jouissance that exceeds reproduction), the death drive is more than sexuality. The death drive includes aggressiveness and death wishes, but the push for the emptiness of Being, is much more than annihilation or extinction.

In my opinion, the way to reconcile the two points of view, that "higher" ethical feelings are cultural acquisitions or that they represent elements of a basic instinctual behavioural repertoire, is to think of the problem in terms of the problems posed by the Freudian theory of sublimation.

Sublimation for Freud represents a cultural acquisition and a healthy form of defence against a primitive drive, and at the same time sublimation represents a direct satisfaction/manifestation of the drive without involving repression. Perhaps Freud never added a paper on sublimation to his metapsychological papers, because of this paradox. "The absence of a coherent theory of sublimation continues to be one of the gaps in psychoanalytic thought" (Laplanche & Pontalis, 1967, p. 417).

Kindness can be a manifestation of both forms of sublimation, either as a reaction formation against hate/greed, or a direct manifestation of the drive in relation to its object. In Seminar VII Lacan (1959–1960) defines sublimation as what elevates the object (the archaic mother) to the dignity of *das Ding*. Now can we really say that *das Ding* represents a direct manifestation of the drive and a direct form of experience?

Satisfaction is also linked to the category of the impossible and the Real as an obstacle, or to the fact that Lacan says that the 'thing' is 'veiled' or 'concealed.' This is not unlike what Lacan has said about the phallus, which is a missing phallus. The object cause of desire appears to be the imaginary phallus, but in fact the signifier of the phallus is a missing phallus, and what the subject is actually looking for is its lack or emptiness, a fact that coincides with the definition of *das Ding* as the veiled presence of a dignified void, and the definition of the drive (and a death drive at that) as a push towards the emptiness of Being (Lacan, 1959–1960, Section X).

Das ding is not a substitutive object of social utility but does not present itself directly either. It presents itself as a dignified void at the centre of the Real around which the subject's sublimity revolves. Satisfaction is a direct satisfaction but only in relationship to a void as a form of jouissance (the 'no-thing').

Kindness, as a function of *das Ding*, represents a form of love in the Real, where what is satisfying is the emptiness of *das Ding*, and it is this emptiness as jouissance that constitutes fondness or kindness for the neighbour as-in-oneself. In the emptiness/lack of the Other, the subject finds its own emptiness/lack, and in the emptiness of the subject, the subject realizes that the emptiness of the Other is the heart's desire.

It is important to differentiate between a defensive or substitutive socially acceptable non-sexual satisfaction, that may preserve some of the intensity of the sexual drive, from how the death drive is a push for the 'no-thing' or *das Ding* embedded within the drive itself.

The push for emptiness is not a teleological principle embedded within the drive and unfolding in stages of development, but rather the satisfaction of circling around the object of the drive without trying to attain it. Attainment is impossible or can only be attained when it is not attained. When effort or will is exerted with a mind free of attainment, then attainment is attained. When jouissance is stopped, another jouissance is attained in its place. Something is attained in the mind of non-attainment or emptiness. In this account, sublimation is not attained by turning sexual libido into ego libido and desexualizing it in the process, but rather by an appeal to something asexual or empty in the nature of the drive itself.

On the one hand, the sexual drive is an instinct aimed at safeguarding the survival of the species through reproduction, and on the other hand, human sexuality in culture acquires characteristics that are not found in animals.

In speaking beings, the sexual drive goes beyond biological reproduction, but the death drive also goes beyond the annihilation or nihilism associated with aggressiveness. Jouissance, as the affective or energetic unity of pleasure and pain represents the interdependency of the sexual and death drives. Jouissance goes beyond reproduction but also goes beyond the fusion with the Other, and the surplus value of phallic jouissance that is always concerned with who has or has not the imaginary phallus. The function of symbolic castration takes the subject from phallic jouissance to the Other or Third jouissance

Regarding the sexual drive in speaking beings, some feminist ethologists (Zihlman, 2012) have argued that sexual activity among some primates can be divorced from reproduction and can take place with partners with whom reproduction is not an option. Supposedly this would free women from reproductive bondage associated with heterosexual sexuality and the patriarchal family organization.

In his drive theory, Freud (1905) used the concept of "anaclisis" (from the Greek relying on, depending on) to account for how the drive is derived from or relies on a biological self-preservation instinct. But just as with the somatic source of the drive, the drive acquires a significant independence once it becomes established within a symbolic/psychical order. The notion of a psychical drive develops out of the prototype of the experience of satisfaction whereby in the process of satisfying biological needs for nutrition and growth, a *jouissance* develops in the infant linked to the satisfaction itself, independent from the needs of the biological organism.

Now this satisfaction remains inextricably linked to the other as *objet a*. The relationship to another subject is more satisfying than autoerotism, for example, because sexuality not only comes from the other, but also is qualified and mediated by the desire of the other. Sexuality becomes inextricably linked with the *objet a* as a remainder of the other within the subject once the other is lost through separation and absence.

Does this feature of human sexuality within culture represent a mechanism of evolutionary change? On the one hand in the Freudian theory of the sexual drive, pleasure becomes independent from biological reproduction, but this does not seem to have a survival value for the individual or the species, or does it?

On the other hand, the very mechanism by which the sexual drive becomes independent from reproduction is the very mechanism by which sexuality becomes regulated by cultural norms rather than biological ones. This allows for increased sexual pleasure while the same pleasure is now regulated by culture rather than biology.

Now does the regulation by culture rather than biology represent a form of evolutionary change? When it comes to the behavioral repertoire of the sexual instinct that is rejected by culture, culture seems to change human sexuality first into the pleasure of the object for its own sake rather than reproduction, and secondarily this feature of the drive is controlled by culture rather than biology.

For Freud, the drive for self-preservation is associated with ego drives that function according to the reality principle and not the pleasure principle defined as the impulse towards hallucinatory wish fulfillment. However, for Freud the pleasure principle is also what regulates defenses to avoid unpleasure and this is the interpretation that Lacan gives of the pleasure principle with the additional caveat that Lacan links the pleasure principle thus defined to the signifier and culture.

The drive towards self-preservation obviously also operates at the level of biological hunger and the self-preservation of the individual as distinct from reproduction/sexuality (the preservation of the species). Once hunger is satisfied and self-preservation is no longer in question, then wish fulfillment arises as the pleasure or frustration of the fantasy object rather than simply the need-satisfying properties of the reality object. The ego, the Preconscious system, and the secondary process all arise to modify the primary process associated with the fantasy object.

The biological drives for nutrition and reproduction are not the same as the processes that emerge to regulate the primary process, and the primary process is not the same as self-preservation as a biological drive. However, the secondary process and reality testing, as efforts to curtail hallucinatory wish fulfillment (primary process), achieve their aims with the support of the drive towards self-preservation.

Thus, the concept of anaclisis applies to both the sexual drive under the pleasure principle, and to the Preconscious and the ego under the reality principle. Biological self-preservation under culture splits or redoubles into non-biological desire and cultural regulation and their mutual determination. In human beings, sexual desire is produced by the interaction of a biological drive and cultural or societal principles. At the same time culture is inseparable from desire as a modified biological instinct within culture that is also in a polarized relationship with culture. Culture modifies biology, but the result is a sexual drive that proves to be more unwieldy or present more challenges than the press of biological drives.

References

Darwin, C. (1859). Chapter VII: Instinct. In *On the Origin of Species by Means of Natural Selection, or the Preservation of Favoured Races in the Struggle for Life*. New York: D. Appleton and Company.

Dawkins, R. (1976). *The Selfish Gene*. Oxford: Oxford University Press.

Freud, S. (1905). *Three Essays on the Theory of Sexuality.* SE, 7, 125–245.

Freud, S. (1913). *Totem and Taboo.* SE, 13, 1–161.

Freud, S. (1915). *Instincts and Their Vicissitudes.* SE, 14, 111–140.

Freud, S. (1917). *Mourning and Melancholia.* SE, 14, 239–258.

Freud, S. (1921). *Group Psychology and the Analysis of the Ego.* New York: Norton & Company, 1959.

Geertz, C. (1973). *The Interpretation of Cultures.* New York: Basic Books.

Hobbes, T. (1994 [1668]). *Leviathan.* Cambridge: Hackett Publishing Company.

Lacan, J. (1992 [1959–1960]). *The Seminar of Jacques Lacan, Book VII: The Ethics of Psychoanalysis* (D. Porter, Trans.). New York: W. W. Norton.

Lamarck, J. B. (1914 [1809]). *Zoological Philosophy.* London: Cambridge University Press.

Laplanche, J. B., & Pontalis, J. B. (2004 [1967]). *Diccionario de Psicoanalisis.* Buenos Aires: Paidos.

Levy-Strauss, C. (1969 [1949]). *The Elementary Structures of Kinship.* Boston: Beacon Press.

MacNeill, A. (2009). *The Complete Works of Charles Darwin Online.* Darwin-online.org. Accessed 29 Aug 2017.

Rose, H., & Rose, S. (2010). Darwin and After. *New Left Review, 63,* 91–113.

Weismann, A. (1889). *Essays Upon Heredity.* London: Oxford Clarendon Press (Full online text available).

Zihlman, A. (2012). The Real Females of Human Evolution. *Evolutionary Anthropology, 21,* 270–276.

3
The Grammatical Voice of the Drive

Lacan (1981/1964) believed the sexual drive to be linked to the unconscious through what he called a nodal point of desire that is not the same as drive. Desire in turn depends on sexual demands articulated in language that always leave a metonymic unsatisfied remainder running under them that Lacan calls desire (p. 154).

This notion of demand, that never completely discharges the tensions associated with desire, Freud locates first in the body, as demands of the body placed upon the mind. Lacan later reinterprets the demands of the body as a social demand or the Other's demand, the demands of the body are interchangeable with the social demands of "the man" or the Other. Something biological and psychical functions through intersubjective interactions and the interactions between need, demand, and desire.

When we dream of food, not having gone to bed hungry, is not purely about the biological need for food. Food objects in such dreams have been sexualized and represent forbidden objects. The oral needs of the body can be sexualized. Sexuality in humans is lived through partial objects and drives apprehended in the network of signifiers. Human sexuality is partial with respect to the biological end of reproduction, even though the partial imaginary and symbolic lures associated with

R. Moncayo, *Knowing, Not-Knowing, and Jouissance*, The Palgrave Lacan Series,
https://doi.org/10.1007/978-3-319-94003-8_3

human sexuality (the signifiers, the sounds, the clothes, the settings, the seduction involving the hidden or revealed parts of the body, etc.), all entice a sexual act that could lead to jouissance just as much as reproduction. In fact, the reproductive and pleasure/pain (jouissance) oriented forms of sexuality also have an inside/outside relationship. What seems like a pursuit of excess can lead to reproduction and what appears to be a bodily sign of reproduction may be a purely sexual and unconsciously fantasized imaginary pregnancy (think of the example of phantom pregnancies).

Following Freud, Lacan stresses that the sexual drive in humans is a myth, a convention, or a fiction. It is in the light of this assumption that he examines the four terms that Freud distinguishes in the drive: the source, the thrust, the object, and the aim.

Thrust is the discharge of an internal quantity of energy or excitation. The needs involved in biological hunger and thirst are also forms of internal excitation and this is also an aspect of the drive of the real ego (not to be confused with Lacan's new ego of the Real) to satisfy the needs of the organism.

But this real ego described by Freud (1895) in the 'Project' (that Lacan defines as a central nervous system regulated by homeostasis or the tendency to realize a balance of internal tensions), is quickly replaced by the pleasure ego and its imaginary objects. To the latter is attributed the task of satisfying the needs of the organism in the form of the object cause of desire. The object of the reproductive sexual drive becomes the object of desire ruled by signifiers. As such the drive also becomes a constant force and not something temporary or rhythmic such as hunger or thirst.

Using the example of sublimation as one of the vicissitudes of the drive, Lacan defines the aim not as pleasure but satisfaction. Then he defines satisfaction by linking it to the category of the impossible and the Real, which is not the opposite or binary negation of the possible. He associates the Real of the drive to its desexualization beyond the biology of need and reproduction. So, does the Real of the drive refer to its desexualization or sexualization beyond the biology of reproduction? Both seem to work at this level. The Real of the drive is something different from both hallucinatory wish fulfillment and the biology of need.

Any object can be used for the purposes of the Real of the drive and not only the object of fantasy or of biological need.

Sublimation is what elevates an object to the dignity of *Das ding*, as Lacan (1959–1960) stated in Seminar VII (Chapter VIII, Section 3). There is something dignified not only in Culture but also in the drive as the no-thing. The drive to elevate an object to the dignity of *das Ding* differs both from the dignity of culture (associated with frustration/castration) or the cultural chaos that can be generated by a biological animal instinct (the primal horde). Sublimation is a direct satisfaction of the drive rather than simply a cultural repressive and substitutive mechanism. In addition, Marcuse (1955) spoke of a repressive de-sublimation that associates the undoing of sublimation, or the unleashing of the primal drives, with repression. The contemporary super ego of late capitalism (neo-liberalism) now demands rather than forbids pleasures, and demanding such pleasures, is a way of repressing the lack or the push towards emptiness associated with desire.

The direct satisfaction of the drive is generated by an impossible relation to a veiled 'thing' or 'no-thing' (*das Ding*) that lies within an enchanted circle from which light ushers forth. *Das Ding* is represented by a void, and the drive from the point of view of sublimation, represents a push towards the emptiness of Being (Lacan, 1959–1960, Section X).

The aim of the drive, what produces enjoyment is simply to move around the object, or to encircle or circumambulate the object rather than reaching the elusive object directly like one would do with an object of social utility. The drive begins in the erogenous zone, circles around the object, and then returns to the erogenous zone. It is in circling around the object, which is an object of the Other, that the drive becomes something else in the cultural field and dimension of the Other.

What Freud means by the vicissitudes of drives refers to the defenses against the drive although the last vicissitude (sublimation) both is and is not a defense. Repression is well known as a defense but the reversal of a drive into its opposite and the turning around upon the subject's own self are freshly treated in Freud's (1915) paper on "*Drives and Their Vicissitudes*". He further notes that reversal of a drive into its opposite involves two different processes: a change from activity to passivity, and a reversal of its content.

The two examples that Freud uses are sadism and masochism and scopophilia or voyeurism and exhibitionism. From looking to being looked at and from love to hate. Thus Lacan (1981/1964) writes:

> Freud now introduces us to the drive by one of the most traditional ways, using at every moment the resources of language, and not hesitating to base himself on something that belongs only to certain linguistic systems, the three voices, active, passive and reflexive. (p. 177)

In language and the Symbolic, the drive circulates around the three grammatical voices of a verb, the actions it describes, and the participants or arguments of the action. The active voice is when the subject is the doer of the action. The passive voice is when the subject is undergoing the action. Not all languages have the middle or reflexive voice in which the subject is both the agent and the receiver or recipient of the action. Some languages have five voices. In the reflexive voice the subject acts on itself as in making oneself seen or heard rather than simply saying the subject is seen or heard. In addition, to these grammatical voices, the vicissitudes of a drive involve the influences of two other polarities: subject-object, and pleasure and pain, or the pleasant and unpleasant.

We observe here the regulation of the drive in the forms of language, where the drive is no longer a solely inherited or genetic instinct. Different codes regulate the genes and the cultural environment in which the sexual drive manifests. Lacan even argues that:

> The passage from the oral drive to the anal drive can be produced not by a process of maturation, but by the intervention of something that does not belong to the field of the drive-by the intervention, the overthrow, of the demand of the Other. (idem, p. 180)

The social Other triggers the movement from phase to phase, and from one zone of the body to another. The weaning from the breast produces a frustration that ends the oral phase of development. The cultural code frustrates or coincides/punctuates the child's readiness to separate from the breast. Lacan points out that the transition from the oral to the anal phase cannot be deduced one from the other or from a biological process of maturation.

What takes place between the oral and anal phases is the inversion of demand, something that will remain a structural feature of the structure of demand. In the oral phase the child and the body demand an amount of work from the parent and the mind. In the anal phase, the demand moves to the side of the parent and the mind who/that demands that the child acquire sphincter control and release feces. There is no continuity between the anal phase and the phallic phase even though breast, feces, and the phallus are all *objet a* and share a place in the unconscious equation.

Feces or excrete is an object of waste meant to be lost and this is another quality of the *objet a* shared with the breast. These are objects meant to be lost under Culture. The loss of a turd begins to prefigure the loss/retention of the phallus and urine under symbolic castration as another form of the negative known as privation and frustration in the oral and anal phases.

The three forms of the negative are intrinsic to the cultural regulation and mediation of the sexual drive. In the phallic phase, what is looked for is not the phallus but its absence. The phallic phase is also organized differently on the side of culture or what Lacan calls the field of the Other. The phallic phase and phallic jouissance, therefore, is regulated by the cultural code and this is what in psychoanalysis is known as symbolic castration.

Lacan also clarifies that the drive is not perverse despite Freud's characterization of the child as polymorphously perverse. The drive is only technically perverse when the subject assumes the place of the object. In the sadistic-masochistic drive the subject makes itself the object of another subject's cruelty.

In the polymorphous perversion of childhood, since in early childhood there is no ego, a child can be both innocent and perverse at the same time, and perverse here has a different natural connotation prior to the distinction between good and bad. An example of this would be when a child upon successful toilet training manages to defecate in the toilet he/she may turn around and gaze at the long and short turds and say the long turd is the mother and the short turd is the child thus reflecting a cloacal theory of reproduction, or a link between sexuality and defecation, and between a turd and a human being. Many of these qualities are also found in sexual perversions.

If the subject knows the good and disavows it, then this is a different matter altogether. In the genital drive the subject is placed according to castration and sexual difference. In perversion, due to the disavowal of sexual difference, the subject assumes the role of the object ($a \rightarrow \$$), while in neurosis the object is what the subject is lacking and looking for in the other ($\$\Diamond a$) who also doesn't have the object.

In his paper, Freud also observes that although love and hate are involved in the sexual drive, love and the sexual drive are heterogeneous or are not made with the same elements. Lacan maps out this distinction unto the other distinction that he made between the phallic drive, and the oral and anal drives. Love and the phallic drive are narcissistic and in the field of the Other, while the oral and anal drives are not. I am not certain this is the case but let the argument stand for the moment as a working hypothesis.

The idea of narcissistic love would collide head on (like particles of matter and antimatter) with the cultural notion of love as something altruistic. Does this mean that egoism and altruism should be an additional vicissitude of the drive when seen from the perspective of love in relationship to the phallic drive? Is love and hate something inevitably narcissistic as reflected in the saying that all is fair in love and war? Lacan writes:

> I suggest that there is a radical distinction between loving oneself through the other-which, in the narcissistic field of the object, allows no transcendence to the object included-and the circularity of the drive, in which the heterogeneity of the movement out and back shows a gap in its interval. (idem, p. 194)

With the oral and anal drives, a gap is revealed between the object of the drive and the source of the drive in the erogenous zone. In narcissistic love, there is no gap due to the illusory completion represented by a subject that has fused and completed itself through the object. The object's transcendence or Otherness has been shut out by the function that the love object has for the subject. But this romantic phase of fusion with the imaginary love object is impermanent and will eventually dissipate. The love for the symbolic Other and for the equality of the Law is something different from the love for the imaginary love object. Is there a form of a so-called mature altruistic object love or a love or knowledge of the Other that is not narcissistic?

The concept of narcissism is broader than how it is defined by an ideology of pure altruistic love that could function as a humanistic ideology or as a defense against narcissism. If anything, the love for the object at the expense of the subject, also takes place in romantic love, or even in war, where the survival of the individual is predicated on the group, and so the defense of the group in that context has priority over the surface preoccupations with the individual. This condition is like relative primary narcissism where the love, identification with, and clinging to the breast is precisely what represents narcissism and the self.

Nonetheless, the love of the Other and being loved by the Other, at work in the ego ideal (the source and agency of values) requires the maturity that comes with the acceptance of the negative and symbolic castration. Maturity and character here means the ability to accept and process a loss and a lack in the subject and in the Other.

The fusion of love with the phallic or genital phase is narcissistic and imaginary while the drive in the oral and anal phases operate in the Real without narcissism. It is unclear in Lacan's text whether this refers to orality and anality per se or just to the oral and the anal rims as erogenous zones of the sexual drive. It is also not clear how hate of the real external environment and the social Other, could remain free of narcissism.

The breast and feces as *objet a* are not devoid of the narcissistic investments associated with the partial object in Freud's (1917) notion of an unconscious equation (phallus, breast, feces, baby, money, gift, etc.). But perhaps Lacan's point is that an adult narcissistic fixation on feces as an *objet a* can only be observed in perversions. The breasts of a woman can serve narcissistic functions for both her and her partner and can also underwrite a mother's omnipotence with respect to her baby's dependence on her breasts. But this is something that takes place in neurosis as well as perversions.

Love of the other as an object, rather than as Other, is first imaginary and narcissistic. For Lacan the object is always a self-object and what is called the total or whole object is not an object but rather the Other. This formulation of the object as other preserves the Freudian notion of the object as a partial psychical object, and at the same time is in accord with the phenomenological, existential, and critical tradition that objects to the objectification of other human beings.

Precisely human beings are no longer objectified when the category of the other/Other is introduced. It is the Other than can mediate between the narcissistic notions of love and hate, and how the object can be both loved and hated at the same time. The object/other is hated when the other represents something more than, or less than the object that the subject or ego is in love with or that serves as the object of desire.

> If for the moment, we define loving as the relation of the ego to its sources of pleasure, the situation in which the ego loves itself only and is indifferent to the external world illustrates the first of the opposites which we found to 'loving'. (Freud, 1915, p. 133)

On the same page, Freud enumerates the opposites of loving in the following order: (1) hating, (2) being loved; and (3) indifference.

For Freud love is on the same side as the ego and both are opposed by the external world and hate. As hate is unpleasant, love is pleasant. Freud then clarifies that the love object and the object of the drive are not the same. For Freud love and hate are examples of the relations of the total ego to objects or to total objects.

Here is where Lacan says that love is imaginary or a relation to the All or the totality of visual perception and that hate or "aggressiveness" is also narcissistic. Love and hate are in relationship to the mirror and to the Other. Although love is narcissistic there is a desire to be loved by the other and to love and hate the self as well. Aggressiveness is also narcissistic given the hate of a frustrating and potentially dangerous external world and given the Other installed at the heart of subjectivity. Both love of self and hate of the Other and the external world are predicated on the totality of the body image that constitute the ideal ego and alter ego behind which lies the Other as mirror that frames the experience of the self-image.

The ideal ego or the specular image as a total image in the mirror is in the place of the Other and therefore the mirror as the cultural Other, and the mother's fantasy object that frames the body image of the child, always threaten the unity of the ego with fragmentation or the shattering of the mirror into its components pieces.

There is a sense of alienation that comes from the fact that the self and body-image are framed by the object and the Other, and the object of the Other's desire. A reflection in the mirror also has a function of reflection/doubt (thinking) that is formative of the body image as a material fact, and as a metaphor.

What can be seen and improved in the mirror and judged as better or worse, refers to both the instrument or reflector (techne) and the image/reflection and its content. Lacan says that there is a blank spot or hole in the image of the body that pushes to be filled to feel whole. But such love of wholeness or totality or the hate of the hole in the image is only imaginary and the trick is to leave the hole empty and be its own fullness.

> It is thus the erectile organ—not as itself, or even as an image, but as a part that is missing in the desired image—comes to symbolize the place of jouissance; this is why the erectile organ can be equated with the $\sqrt{-1}$, the symbol of the signification produced above, of the jouissance it restores—by the coefficient of its statement—to the function of the missing signifier: (−1). (Lacan, 1960 [2006], p. 307)

In fact, this is what happens in development given that the hole is filled by the search for an alter ego who could be the mother's perfect *objet a* before the search moves on to the development of the ego ideal and the search for the father or the paternal function that will embody symbolic castration. From then on castration will be symbolized as sexual difference. A woman is desired because she is the phallus and what makes her be the phallus, or the object of desire, is that she lacks the penis (idem, p. 310). What is desired about the phallus is its absence as a penis.

Lacan says that in the blank spot in the image, even the zero as a concept of absence, and the absence of an object, is missing. Inside the blank spot/hole Lacan finds the square root of –1 ($\sqrt{-1}$) which is an imaginary number that is not a real number and does not exist although as an imaginary number it can be placed in the line of real numbers to generate complex numbers. The love for self, the love for the ideal ego, and the association of the blank spot with the genitals is what undergirds, according to Lacan, the connection that Freud noted between love, genital love, and drive.

Both femininity and the phallus are numbers that do not exist and yet can be used as operands to produce sense and different levels of meaning. The phallus for Lacan is a missing signifier and in Seminar XI (1964) he says that this is what we are looking for more than the phallus. The phallus as a lack is also descriptive of femininity and in fact the lack is what both sexes have in common.

Lacan says that the symbol for the null set (Ø), or the imaginary number (i or $\sqrt{-1}$) emerges out of the place and symbol of the symbolic phallus as a missing phallus or an empty place of substitution, a structuring gap within the Symbolic. Masculine lack is symbolized by the symbolic phallus while feminine lack is symbolized by the square root of –1.

Lacan then applies the passive grammatical voice of the drive (of 'making oneself'the object of an action) in such a way that the absence of the phallus is concretized into its invagination represented by the square root of $\sqrt{-1}$. Either the vagina or the penis can be represented as the desired presence or absence of the phallus. The vagina is fucking itself with a phallus produced by evagination, or turning the vagina inside out, or the phallus is fucking itself in its own sheath or by invagination or turning the phallus outside in and pushing it back into the body. Here the drive works with body parts, part object symbolization, and organ pleasure, and the ego as a totality disappears.

Love characterizes the relation of the total ego to its sexual objects and Freud clarifies that love here cannot begin until the tender feelings towards the object are fused with the primacy of the genitals. Such fusion works in the service of the reproductive function that only begins with biological maturation at the time of puberty. Romantic love and the diffusion of self-other boundaries that it implies, is what covers over the differences between the sexes, enacts the instinct for self-preservation (of the species), and justifies the tendency for a personal and pleasure-based satisfaction (the good of pleasure as distinct from the pleasure of the good).

Freud says that love begins with self-love or narcissism or the capacity to obtain pleasure from auto-eroticism and organ pleasure self-referentially defined. Then from narcissism, love passes over to the object but the object here is not a symbolic other but simply a narcissistic object that the ego appears to lack and the other appears to have.

The object of desire disrupts the reciprocity between loving and being loved, because the subject may love but not be loved or may be loved but not love the other in a romantic or sexual way. In such cases, romantic love may turn into hating either the ego or the other in the external world.

The fusion between self and other, and between tenderness and sex drive or the object of the drive, takes place counter-intuitively not between two subjects but between the fantasy objects of two subjects. However, since there is a rift or a gap between the fantasy object and the other, the fantasy object will inevitably fall and change and be lost in some way.

Lacan argues that in love the subject is fundamental, but this is not the same as the ego. He links the gaze to the Symbolic and the subject, in the same way that the theory links the recognition and naming of the ideal ego, or its symbolic ratification, to the gaze of the father and the Name as a unary trait. The gaze of the father functions as a transitional *objet a* between the ideal ego and the ego ideal. Both the gaze of the mother and the gaze of the father help establish the scopic drive in the subject.

It is in the gaze or the scopic drive that Lacan finds desire, the subject, and the Symbolic order, their interactions with the sexual drive, and the place where love and sex are fused. Love and the gaze interact with the genital drive by covering the genitals and relating to them through the clothing assigned/generated by the symbolic order.

The signifier is what represents and substitutes. Lacan also says that the cycle of birth and death substitutes and represents immortal life and at the same time through representation a remainder is generated of what was lost of immortal life in sexual reproduction.

With representation, there is something of the represented that is lost. The S_1 that is S_0 is lost when S_1 becomes S_2. There is something of immortal life that is lost with the placenta as a symbol of fusion and reproduction. Then with birth a substitute to the placenta is generated in the form of the baby's relationship to the breast, and the placenta itself will be lost. The breast will acquire the qualities of the placenta and immortal life until the breast itself is lost with weaning.

But at this point the subject will have already emerged as a signifier in the field of the Other. The subject is born in so far as the signifier emerges in the field of the Other. The subject is lost behind the signifier, in the same way that immortal life and the placenta are lost behind the breast or the object. This double loss of the subject and the object, that connects the two as presence or absence in the field of the drive and the field of the Other (as a social subject that is also the subject of the drive), is what creates the space to link signifiers to their objects, the phallus to the *objet a*, and the coupling of organs.

Loss of immortal life, of the placenta, the *objet a* and the phallus, makes death present within the sexual drive as Lacan (1960 [2000]) says, as well as how in death the subject may wish to recover immortal life, and the *objet a*.

> In this way I explain the essential affinity of every drive with the zone of death, and reconcile the two sides of the drive-which, at one and the same time, makes present sexuality in the unconscious and represents, in its essence, death. (p. 199)

For Lacan, it is the gaze that joins the subject of the drive and the subject in the field of the Other and in the process, love may prevail over hate in relationship to the Other. However, since love according to Freud and Lacan is narcissistic and narcissism in relationship to the Other and the external world leads to hate, I am not sure how love and life could gain the upper hand over hate and death at least during a person's life.

Since the scopic drive and the gaze as an *objet a* link up with the object that represents immortal life or death among the world of living objects, another way of saying the same thing is that the gaze wants to see the unseen or the very visage of death, inherent emptiness, and immortal life amid the object world.

Of course, it is at this point, that the Other, in so far as it substitutes and represents immortal life and its loss, as the original form of loss, becomes the figure not only of the life that is possible within culture, but also of death itself. Death and the death drive here appear to win over the aggressiveness that bears the mark of narcissism. In so doing, the Other as death may push the limits of love beyond narcissism.

References

Freud, S. (1895). *A Project for a Scientific Psychology. The Standard Edition of the Complete Psychological Works of Sigmund Freud* (Vol. 1, pp. 283–397). London: Hogarth Press.

Freud, S. (1915). *Instincts and Their Vicissitudes*. SE, 14, 111–140.

Freud, S. (1917). *On Transformations of Instinct as Exemplified in Anal Eroticism* (J. Strachey, Trans.). SE, 17, 127–133.

Lacan, J. (1960 [2006]). The Subversion of the Subject and the Dialectic of Desire. In *Ecrits* (B. Fink, Trans). New York: Norton.

Lacan, J. (1981 [1964]). *The Four Fundamental Concepts of Psychoanalysis*. New York: Norton.

Lacan, J. (1992 [1959–1960]). *The Seminar of Jacques Lacan: The Ethics of Psychoanalysis, Book VII*. New York: Norton.

Marcuse, H. (1955). *Eros and Civilization*. New York: The Beacon Press.

4

Signs, Objects, Icons (Images), Indexes, Representamen/Representations, Interpretants, and Habit in the Work of Peirce and in the Light of Lacanian Theory

A core idea behind Peirce's understanding of the relationship between a concept and an object is that the content of a concept is revealed in the effects that the concept has on the object. As Peirce (1867) put it, 'our conception of these effects is the whole of our conception of the object' (Essential Peirce (EP), Vol. 1, p. 132).

Whether the concept determines the object or the object determines the concept, the least we can say is that the concept and the object arise together or mutually determine each other. Concepts are embedded in the perception of the object to the same extent that language is unconscious or constitutes the background of perception. A subject perceives the meaning of an object but thinks the meaning arises from the object because the faculty of Sense, that determines the meaning of the object, is unconscious in a descriptive sense. The unconscious symbolic structure is experienced as a conscious relationship to the object and the actions performed in relationship to the object. This is what is pragmatic about Peirce's approach except that the unconscious symbolic structure has an existence of its own independently from the actions performed by a subject in relationship to an object in the external world.

R. Moncayo, *Knowing, Not-Knowing, and Jouissance*, The Palgrave Lacan Series,
https://doi.org/10.1007/978-3-319-94003-8_4

Language is unconscious or empty from the point of view of the perceiving subject. What the subject perceives instead is the naïve reality of the object. In the naïve perception of an object we have the object, the sense organ used, and the consciousness/interpretation of the object. The concept is embedded in the meaning provided by the faculty of 'sense' rather than the sense organ. Another way of saying it, is that the concept can be found embedded in the meaning assigned to the object. Consciousness and the mind here are equivalent to the faculty of Sense as meaning and, in this respect, the mind is larger than consciousness.

For Peirce the interpretant or interpretation of a sign/representation is a second representamen or representation. The first or primary representation for Peirce represents an object, the meaning of which is given by a second representation/signifier.

For Peirce, the object and the interpretant are two correlates of the sign; the one being antecedent, the other consequent of the sign. The problem with Peirce's theory of the sign is that it conceives of an original relation between the sign/representation and the object, as if the sign had derived from a quality of the object instead of the signifier determining the meaning of the object world.

For Lacan the early form of the signifier, in the form of the unary trait, tally, or letter, is derived from the object but not from a part of the object that is represented by the sign, as Peirce believed, but from the quality of the object, that originally represented the death or killing of an animal as a source of food. An initial mark or unary trace/number represented the dead animal. From these early marks/letters, systems of numbers and letters would evolve.

For example the letter a, the aleph, or the first letter of the alphabet is said to represent the icon of the head of a cow, bull, steer, or bovine specimen, turned upside down. That is, take the head of a cow and turn it upside down and you have some form of the letter A. This example seems to corroborate Peirce's idea that the sign takes and represents a part of the object that in this case represents a source of food or nutrition.

However, with a letter we have a sign but not a system of signs. The order of the structure requires the repression/forgetting of the iconic origins of letters in order for letters to constitute words and phrases or statements. The place of the origin is replaced by the void left by the absence of the object. Thus Lacan described the primal object or *objet a* as the index of a void. In this case the index does not refer to the proximity/contiguity or similarity with the object. Proximity in this sense does not point to the physical presence of the object but rather to the subjective proximity of the object in light of its absence.

A symbol represents the absence/death/loss of the life-giving object. Death or the unmarked behind the symbolic system is what “kills” the direct or immediate link between a sign and its object. The mark or unary trace at the origin of language or a symbolic system, is a mark of the unmarked and the unmarked represents what is left behind of the unmediated relation to the object world. From then on what we call objects are signifiers within language that construct the images of the world. The immediate reference to the object is not through the signifier or the cultural object but through the unmarked.

The unmarked comes to occupy the empty place of a placeholder function that will facilitate various types of relations among numbers and signifiers. Once a symbolic system has emerged the sign will represent a signifier/signified relation that will define the nature of the object.

According to psychoanalysis or a psychoanalytic use of the concept of a Symbolic order or language, the meaning of objects is defined by the signifier in its relation to the iconic representation of the object. The signifier also emerges from the field generated by the loss of the object. The relationship to objects and the object world is mediated by anterior losses of the object that mark the object with the mark of a lack and the lack represents not only the potential loss of the object but also the mark of the unmarked defined as either what lies beyond representation (true hole) or the mark of the killing of the object that has been denied (false hole).

The current relation to the object and the object world is mediated by the signifier. Peirce naively considers that the original relation to the object has been preserved (its death has been denied) and therefore the representation or the representamen in the present directly mirrors or reflects the object. However, in psychoanalysis meaning is not given by the icon of the object as a component of the sign, but by the second signifier that acts as interpretant for the object. The signifier determines the object world as well as the limits beyond which the beyond the signifier can be found.

However, this beyond the signifier can represent something beyond representation and beyond the Code as the representative of the representation, or it can also point to phenomena regulated by signs/codes that are not linguistic or cultural-symbolic.

For Peirce feelings in themselves outside their verbal components are physiological interpretants but this is not so for Lacan who considers feelings as mediated by the larger Code that regulates the mother-infant relationship. Drives are known through ideational representative representations of objects and through affects that refer to the quantitative or energetic aspect of the representation that represents the drive. Representations not only represent drives, and interact with jouissance, but also represent the Code that regulates the representational system (as the representative of the representation). Condensation and displacement, metaphor and metonymy, work for both the drive and the cultural code.

Before I delve into the examination of the codes involved in what Peirce calls semiosis, or the field of semiotics, and how it differs from Lacan's psychoanalytic concept of a symbolic order, I will first examine and define the concept of Code and its various meanings.

What Is a Code

A code is a system of words, letters, or other symbols substituted for other words, letters, symbols, especially for the purposes of secrecy. Secrecy in psychoanalysis means the same as repression and censorship, and is something that happens automatically, unconsciously, and systematically. Repression works by producing a substitute. Socially, a code is a systematic collection of laws that govern the political and public life of a nation state. Ultimately a subject represses in identification with social norms/codes, despite the fact that repression can also be triggered by physiological mechanisms associated to homeostasis and the pleasure-unpleasure principle.

In either case, whether at the level of the individual, the subject or internal world, or at the level of society and the objective external world, a code restricts and regulates norms, what is acceptable or inadmissible, prescribing how and what to think, and ways to dress and act in society. Alternatively, a code can be a key (or set of instructions) for translating a message. A code can be something non-linguistic such as the telegraph using a system of electrical signals to represent letters or numbers in transmitting messages.

In computer science, a source code is the version of software as it is originally written (i.e., typed into a computer) by a human in plain text. A code can also be an access code such as the code needed to obtain banking and financial information. It can also refer to the genetic code that specify the genes and how the different combinations of the four letters of the genetic code produce a trait, organ, or characteristic: a gene that codes for blond hair, or the formation of wings, instead of arms or legs, for example.

When language brings attention to the code upon which speech depends, the function of the code is considered to be metalinguistic. So, there is no metalanguage, as Lacan says, in the sense of a second language that grounds a first one, but there is something metalinguistic in the existence of the code itself although the code by itself does not have meaning within language. The code has no meaning although the absence of meaning, not as a positive content that has been repressed, can precipitate the movement and transformation of signification.

Semiosis, Habits of Action, and the Sign as a Triadic Relation

Semiosis meant for Peirce something more than language. It could mean any action of a force whether physical or psychical, so that action or force may not be mental or a state of consciousness. By mental, Peirce meant consciousness and therefore the unconscious in this model can be confused with physical and physiological processes.

The sign for Peirce is not an element of the hermeneutic circle like it was for Dilthey, Heidegger, or Gadamer, the continental German philosophers. From this point of view the sign may not be a cultural phenomenon at all. The action of pair-wise relations whether in genetics, between particles, or between cells, would all be semiosis from this point of view. When this view is transferred to behavioral psychology then a sign would be a stimulus for instinctual behavior such as eating that would represent the interpretant of the sign.

The relation between physical/biological signs and cultural signs can be described as the relation between semiotics and linguistics. The field of semiotics refers to the communication of any message writ large, while the field of linguistics is restricted to the communication of verbal messages. The relation between semiotics and linguistics raises the possibility that letters, words, and sentences (the unit levels of the signifier) could serve as connecting links to semiotic signs within the physiological organism.

In Lacanian terms this would be one example of the signifier functioning within the dimension of the Real. Here we have something more than a relation between two signifiers S_1 and S_2 within language. S_0 or $S_1 - S_0$ is a case where the signifier S_0 is in the Real. This signifier functions as a placeholder link at the boundary between two or more sign systems. In the case of the human Symbolic, according to Lacan, the placeholder function is the phallic function itself as the function of symbolic castration. The square root of -1, as well the null set, appear in the place of the missing symbolic phallus. The null set is an index of the Real as the no-code, no law, or no-representation.

With the signifier or the signified in the Real, in the sense of the organism, could we say, for example, that a chain of signifiers/representations is analogous to a chain of neurons? Isn't this just incorrect thinking by analogy? In the field of biological semiotics von Uexküll (1987) proposed the concept of homomorphy to describe a fundamental principle that recurs at different levels of complexity. The concept of homomorphy is similar to Dawkins' concept of replication and meme mentioned in Chapter II. Memes are little pieces of "me" and memory obtained through imitation (identification). Memes represent the homomorphic principle at the level of the mind, more than the brain.

The relation between signifier and signified is an example of a homomorphic replicating principle. Von Uexküll distinguished between a meaning-carrier and a meaning utilizer. A meaning-carrier is an object, whether mental or physical, that carries or is represented by a sign/signifier for another meaning utilizer that in this case would be another subject/signifier. The signifier and the signified are also in a sensor-effector, and sender-receiver form of homomorphy, or replicator relationship, according to von Uexküll's framework.

In this respect, an interesting comparison can be made between Lacan's Symbolic order and von Uexküll's homomorphic principle as the fundamental plan or elementary code that organizes variation or differentiations among signifiers. For von Uexküll, each sign is a variation or differentiation of a binary between self and non-self.

For Lacan the relation between lover and beloved, hunter and prey, man and woman, leads to a freedom resulting from different levels of self and non-self, having and not having, being and non-being. For Lacan the ± in the phallic function is an interplay between having or not having, being or not being the imaginary, fantasized object cause of desire. This is resolved with symbolic castration that opens up a new or different space for desire and its object. Symbolic castration is an example of the non-self replicator at a different Symbolic level.

Lacan made an equivalence between signifier and subject. The pre-subject or the unbarred subject is S. The division of the subject is represented as $ that in turn represents the appearance of two signifiers: S_1 and S_2. S as the first signifier also represents the imaginary phallus that the child is for the mother and that after the phallic symbolic function is represented as the S_2 of the Name of the Other.

Peirce says both things about interpretants: they can be conceived of as being and not being a mental mode (Peirce 1940, p. 275) or modifications of consciousness (EP, Vol. 2, pp. 411–412). I argue that this contradiction in Peirce refers to two different modalities: the Semiotic or Semiosis and the Symbolic. Both modalities respond to different codes that are also in relationship with each other. The semiotic or semiosis is not mental while the Symbolic is. In addition, *lalangue* or the language of the Real unconscious does not have a Code like the structure of language, which is unconscious in a descriptive sense.

In contrast to Kristeva's (1941) semiotic, that appears to distinguish between maternal and paternal, pre-oedipal and oedipal languages, *lalangue* does refer to the desire of the mother but does not have its own Code, the way the Symbolic does. In addition, semiosis or the semiotic in Peirce does have very specific codes that are not Symbolic or Cultural but have symbolic effects, nonetheless, as well as vice versa. Researching this question further may result in interesting practical applications to the field of psychosomatic phenomena.

Kristeva also links the semiotic to the musical and the poetic, however, in Lacan the beyond language, jouissance or the Real, is also included in the Borromean knot (RSI) together with the Symbolic and the Imaginary. The structure of music and sound (the amplitude of the wave, for example) is entirely mathematical, yet sound and the voice, as an *objet a*, with its tone, pitch and loudness, points to the Real beyond the signifier. The senseless Real is without Law or Code, yet interacts with both. Now does the desire of the mother have any independence outside the Name of the Father or does the NoF overdetermine the desire of the mother? Does the Real have independence from the Symbolic or does the Symbolic determine the Real? Well the answer is both.

In Lacan's paternal metaphor $\frac{NoF}{Desire\ of\ Mother}$ the desire of the mother as a signified is represented by the object cause of desire itself represented by the signifier of the imaginary phallus, and at the same time the desire of the mother is the signified for a signifier of jouissance (NoF) without another signifier as the signified, since the signifier is in the Real. In the latter case, the Real and the desire of the mother is beyond symbolic/phallic signification. However, here there is a difference pointing to the pre/trans phallacy. The totalizing bond between the mother and the child, as reflected in the jouissance of the (m) Other, has to become a phallic jouissance, that itself then is transformed into a Third jouissance known as the Other jouissance. Only with the other two does the totalizing bond of the jouissance of the Other, become something more than simply being an engulfing inconvenient jouissance.

In Plato the Chora is a Third, as a gap or space/interval between being and non-being, that according to Kristeva supposedly avoids or is beyond the Symbolic. From this perspective, she reduces Lacan's theory to the Oedipal and phallocentric. However, this only applies to the period in Lacan's thought that was focused on the Symbolic. In Seminar XXIII Lacan (1975–1976) says that the Real is the Third that ties the other two registers together rather than the Symbolic. The Real "ex-sists" so it is beyond being and non-being and thus corresponds to the idea of a structuring rather than disruptive gap in relationship to the Symbolic (Moncayo, 2017). Lacan's ideas kept evolving in response to his critics yet without mentioning them by name, as was his policy.

Peirce also recognizes that in human beings at least, semiosis requires the interaction or cooperation of three subjects. The Third here would represent the cultural environment. The modifications of consciousness would be linked to the Third and the cultural environment. It is unclear how the Third would function within the physical dimension other than when the physical functions as an effect or a physiological interpretant of a cultural representation/signifier.

The symbolic or representational system both in Freud and Pierce involve modifications of mind-consciousness. But of course here a theory and an experience of mind-consciousness is required to understand how a symbol impacts mind consciousness. According to Freud (as presented in Chapter 1) there are different types and energetic qualities of representations across the Pcpt-Cs; the Pcs.-Cs.; and Pcs-Ucs. systems that constitute and determine the symbolic structure of the psyche.

Peirce describes the effects that concepts have on the object in terms of habits of action that in humans enact beliefs and practices in relationship to an object. Concepts and signifiers involve habits of action and this is another way that Pierce defines an interpretant, that is to say, the effect that a signifier or an $S_1 - S_2$ relation has on actions and the interaction with objects of social reality and utility.

A habit is both an interpretant and another signifier. Instead of an unconscious signifier/representation having an impact on the body or on the discipline of the body, where the rubber hits the road for the signifier, where it functions, according to Pierce, is on habit as a basic unit of action and behavior.

However, habit in Peirce also comes closer to the experience of psychoanalysis when he considers habit as a form of motivational disposition, whether inborn, innate, or acquired. Habit energies, as motivational dispositions or drives, can be described as interpretants for inscriptions and representations.

> …"habit or disposition," that is, as some general principle working in a man's nature to determine how he will act, then an instinct, in the proper sense of the word, is an inherited habit, or in more accurate language, an inherited disposition. (1940, p. 123)

On the one hand, habit represents a drive, or an inherited disposition, and on the other hand, habit is a set of actions (behaviors) and functions that are acquired in culture rather than inherited. The latter would correspond to the concept of cognitive ego functions within ego psychology and psychoanalysis. Realistic ego functioning coincides with good habits or discipline, in terms of study, health, love, food, sex, etc. Conversely, bad habits would correspond with subjective drives and impulses that are in conflict with the norms of the culture. Examples of these could be addictions, sleep problems, sexual perversions, over-eating, poor hygiene, disheveled appearance, poor handling of money, and various kinds of acting out behavior.

In Peirce's theory the sign relation is a triadic relation. Whenever the representing relation has an instance, we find one thing (the "object") being represented by or stuffed into/embedded within another thing (the "representamen/sign") and being represented to a third thing (the "interpretant"/signified). Moreover, the object is represented by the representamen in such a way that the interpretant is also a representamen of the object to yet another interpretant.

In the three moments of the sign/signifier a thing is found that can be represented by either one of the three. This is similar to Lacan saying that the three circles of the Borromean knot are all self-similar circles as a form of iteration. However, each circle has a different function of equivalence (not identity) in the knot. The thing as object in Freud and Lacan is represented by the Imaginary rather than by an empirical reference. The object in the Imaginary is an icon or more accurately: the thing is an object in the Imaginary. The object is equivalent to the image, and the image becomes equivalent to a thing representation that becomes equivalent to a signifier within a signifying body, and finally the signifier becomes the equivalent of a Code as the representative of the representation. The Code is the final interpretant or Other as the battery or system of signifiers.

Semiosis, the Ideal-Ego, the Unary Trace, and the Symbolic Order

I will now visit the example of the specular image and the mirroring actions of a mother with her infant as used by Muller (1996) in his developmental semiotics wherein he combines Pierce's semiotics with the understanding of psychological development according to psychoanalytic and Lacanian theory.

Muller begins by pointing that interactions between mother and child are mediated by the symbolic code organized by semiosis. Although he wants to use Lacanian theory, Muller uses Pierce's concept of the Third instead of Lacan's notion of the NoF as a representative of the code or the symbolic order. Muller (1996) says that

> the mother's smiling gaze functions for the infant as a sign, as an icon of the infant's smiling gaze as well as an index whose contiguous object is her recognizing presence and whose dynamic interpretant is the infant's smiling gaze in response. (p. 44)

For Muller and Pierce the smile is both an icon and an index of her proximity. In Lacanian theory the gaze of the mother as an *objet a* represents a sign or an icon for the infant. We have said that an icon or an image already requires symbolization but what symbolization could the infant use before language?

The smiling image of the mother and the mirroring of her smile in the infant's smile, represent desire and the desire of the mother as an interpretant. This echoes Lacan's view that desire is the signified of the NoF acting as a signifier. The child sees himself/herself as an icon reflected in the gleam in the mother's eye and the mother's smile as an icon of what gives the mother joy, meaning the infant. Now what is the relation among the icon/image, the object, and the signifier?

The icon is the image of the mother's smile, as a part of the mother as an object, but the question is whether the code rather than the object makes the icon? How are signifiers stuffed into the icon in such a way that determines the meaning of the icon? In addition, how is the contiguity/proximity or the separation from the object factor in as an index of the sign?

The child knows separation from the mother before the smiling response that begins around three months of age. The infant already separated from the body of the mother and already has had the experience of separating from the breast or the experience of the temporary absence of the breast. The body of the mother has been lost and regained with the breast only to be lost once again. The absence of the object has to figure into the process of semiosis and representation.

However, the presence of the mother as an object alternates with her absence and the symbolization of the absence. So how does the icon of her face function as a representation of both her absence and presence? The smile represents the joy of the experience of satisfaction and signals its return after an experience of privation/frustration experienced with anger and/or grief. Thing representations in Freud consist of an energetic investment of images associated with the object and are mostly unconscious. The specular image or the mirroring between mother and child is not unconscious, and the image in the mirror or the ideal ego remains as a life long structure of the subject. What is unconscious is how the Other remains embedded in the image, behind it as it were.

In Peirce's model of semiosis, whether the icon represents the existence of the mother as an object or the index is a measure of her proximity in space, both icon and index point to the mother's presence rather than her absence. Only with the representamen and its interpretation (symbol) is there a choice of representing the mother's absence.

In Lacanian theory the image or icon is already stuffed with the signifier and the unary trace represents presence and absence, proximity and distance. The icon represents the joy of reunion after separation or the risk of separation and its symbolization. But a key point is that the signifier in the mother and father's words is already functioning even before the child learns to speak. In fact, it is the signifier that is given to the child to help mediate and symbolize loss and absence within experience.

Sense, Logic, Number, and Code

Frege (1892) proposed the concept that Sense as signification is a function: (S[ ]). The empty parentheses is used as a placeholder for a particular variable that Frege calls the argument for a mathematical function or the meaning/sense function in language. Whatever indeterminate x is introduced as input into the Sense function produces the value/signifier of the function for argument x.

In mathematics, a function is a precise relation between the elements of a set, for example the set of real numbers, and the elements of another set made of the squares of all the real numbers. Each number as input will be related to its square as output. In this example the mathematical function is x^2 or every number multiplied by itself. A function that relates terms is an operation that structures the relations between terms. A function 'machine' (an oven, for example) takes an object as input (dough) and turns it into a different object (bread) as output. The function transforms dough into bread. There is nothing about a function that implies it must deal with numbers. Any collection of objects will serve as domain and codomain.

Now what about a propositional function within language? A proposition is a statement with a variable that becomes a proposition when the variable is given a value or meaning. Can the Sense function of the Censor function or transform one word or variable into a different word? The Sense function uses signifiers as variables or input and transforms signifiers into signifieds or meaning as output.

The function of Sense in language is how the relation between signifiers produces meaning via the signifier-signified relation. An application of these concepts to psychoanalysis would understand function, for example, as the Censor function of replacing censored meanings within a variable/signifier into socially accepted meanings and signifieds. The function is what erases one signifier and replaces it with another.

Meaning is achieved by a relationship and a function of substitution between signifying elements. A sentence is not a statement until the meaning of a variable is produced. A sentence has to be construed according to the formal rules of grammar and sintax and at the same time its content or signified must conform to socially produced acceptable meaning. The gap in the placeholder function is not closed until a value is produced that can close the meaning of the sentence. Yet the empty value of the placeholder function is never completely closed and the sentence can be ambiguous and suggest more than one meaning or even no-meaning at all.

It is important to note here that the application of a mathematical concept/model to psychoanalysis is no longer mathematics in the strict sense of the term. Some people would be justified in saying 'this is not real mathematics'! It is certainly true that from the point of view of arithmetic or numeric relations, non-algebraic mathematics is not mathematics.

However, numbers are also concepts and others could argue that without the conceptual aspect of mathematics, mathematics could be reduced to computations that can be better performed by computers. In any case, mathematical concepts can be regarded as logical forms although mathematics it is not entirely reducible to logic. In logic, variables are not numbers but the truth-values true and false, represented by 1 and 0, respectively.

Sense is a function that relates one signifier to a second signifier that thanks to the function becomes the meaning of the first. Sense is a function at work in language. A signifier is entered in the function that will produce a value for this signifier within the function of signification. The function of Sense is empty until a signifier is introduced and the combination of the function and the signifier S_1 produces a second signifier as the Sense of the first signifier.

But how does the Sense function relate to the Code as an interpretative framework? The concept of the Code adds the function of censorship/secrecy to the function of Sense as if the function of Sense could be read as either a function of revealing the meaning of S_1 or concealing S_1 with S_2. The concept of Code as Censor is how Sense can be interpreted as a function of censorship/concealment. The Code is an aspect of the unrepressed unconscious, and represents Lacan's attempt to formulate the Freudian concept of the unrepressed unconscious that cannot be reduced to the unrepressed Id.

Sense and Code share the empty parenthesis that allows for the substitution of a variable/signifier S_1 by another (S_2) value given by the function. The substitution, however, is not always for purposes of secrecy or concealment. The substitution of signifiers could also be for purposes of classification such as the genetic code, the codes used for medical diagnoses and their treatments, or the codes used to program computers. The value of the function can also be expressed in sounds, light flashes, or flags, as units of signification based on the sign rather than the signifier.

The input for the Sense function does not have to be numbers or words/signifiers, they could also be sound waves or light waves that are interpreted in terms of concepts or actions. For example, where the sign is not a signifier but a concrete object like a traffic light, the changing light colors are the inputs of the object, that are transformed into actions as outputs or signified: stop or go, on or off. Now the colors could also be metaphors such as green representing the movement and growth of life, while red represents stopping and staying still and away from danger. Now we are in the domain of signifiers, metaphors, and the Symbolic, rather than simply an order of pair-wise relations within a semiotic system of signs.

The function of the Code has a wider application than the function of Sense and Censorship in language, and can refer more widely to the codes that regulate patterns and structures in nature. So there is a connection between Sense and Code where in language Code refers to the function of the Censor or repression at work in metaphor and substitution in language. But there is also the connection between Sense and Code in the 'sense' of sense or non-sense in mathematics.

Sense can refer to meaning, or to sensing the differences between the various sense mediums through which we perceive the world, or it can refer to the symbolic structure and Culture or how social Law regulates language and vice versa. Finally, sense can refer to the function of sense in mathematics. Substitution here functions numerically. We make sense of and control the world by using an abstract world of numbers.

There are hidden (read substitutions) connections between numeric patterns/structures, and not new words or new numbers produced by the function, but the phenomenal descriptions and elements or shapes found in biological forms and their variations, or in planetary orbits and processes, etc. Instead of words, now we have worlds (astronomical, sub-atomic, molecular, viral, genetic, biological). There are indeed numbers and logical connections embedded in biological forms. Since for Freud, the Id was a biological substratum, perhaps he was wrong when in 1933 he said that "The logical laws of thought do not apply in the id and this is true above all of the law of contradiction" (the New Introductory Lectures (SE, 22, p. 73).

The truth value of Freud's statement regarding the Id belongs to the logical level of impulse as experienced by a subject in society. A subject may follow the directives of the laws of desire (I want what I don't have and don't want what I have), or the law of the biological organism (hunger for example), but the equations for these latter two conflict with the equation of what constitutes logical action in society (to use a trivial yet relevant example: to pee (p) or not pee (-p) in public).

There are numbers and logic at work in irrationality and irrational numbers despite the fact that what those numbers may represent in action may contradict what society considers logical according to other perhaps equally mathematical criteria. The irrational is not irrational but rather refers to a different form of rationality that denies the first and vice versa.

For example, the inside is the inside, and the outside is the outside, yet the outside can go inside, and the inside can go outside. Finally, there is a logic or a non-logical order where inside while being inside is neither inside or outside, and outside, while being outside, is neither outside or inside. These three logical dimensions correspond to Lacan's three registers: Dual Imaginary, Non dual Symbolic, and the neither dual nor non-dual Real that is outside the inside-outside distinction.

It is not the case that there is a logical system facing or interacting with another non-logical emotional system (this is only true at a phenomenological or existential human level). Rather it is a matter of different logical types or levels, different levels of negation and of contradiction and non-contradiction. It is not a question of negation and no-negation or a denial of negation, it is a matter of different forms of negation: unary and binary.

In unary negation the negated remains unmarked thus giving off the impression that 'nothing' has been negated. An act or a representation has been negated, and the void or absence left in its wake, can also be negated or replaced with a new representation. What was negated is unconscious and the unconscious appears as a void or a false hole, that itself can be negated. In a unary negation, what is negated is repressed or void, while in a binary negation, the negated is intellectually and consciously accepted.

Things can be perceived as numbers or sound waves, as music or noise, as pleasant or harsh. A harsh sound may produce a so-called irrational response such as fight or flight, attack or defend, and this may contradict a harmonious or pleasant response to sound, but in either case a sound wave will be involved that under certain numeric conditions may produce contradictory or non-contradictory results.

As I have stated elsewhere, the principle of contradiction, as is commonly called, is the logical principle of non-contradiction. Here there seems to be an identity between two opposites or between the name of a relation and its function. Reality is contradictory and the function of rational thought is to separate the true from the false. Existentially, a person appears as either dead or alive, a man or a woman. The law of non-contradiction allows the true statement to be differentiated from the false.

In dreams, however, a male may appear as a woman, and the dreamer may appear alive and yet in the dream not know that they are dead. The dream accepts contradiction while waking life rejects it. The principle of contradiction rejects contradiction and so does the principle of non-contradiction. In this sentence two opposites (contradiction and non-contradiction) paradoxically appear to be identical.

I say paradoxically because the definition of the principle says that opposite propositions cannot be both true, yet the way the principle is named seems to contradict its definition. The principle of non-contradiction obviously rejects contradictions but the principle of contradiction by its very name appears to accept contradiction when in fact it is often used to represent the opposite. Thus, it is clearer to call the principle of contradiction the principle that accepts contradictions, and the principle of non-contradiction, the principle that rejects contradictions.

The law of non-contradiction is the law that creates duality by forbidding different things to be one thing. In contrast to this, the law of contradiction allows opposite or distinct things to be one thing and thus represents a principle of non-duality. By allowing contradiction or duality, the law of contradiction paradoxically eliminates contradiction and duality.

There is no contradiction between saying that there is no object, and that only the subject exists (because the object is defined within the mind/categories of the subject), and saying the opposite: that there is no subject, and that only the object exists (objects of mind define who and what the subject is). In this example, categories of mind (signifiers or names) are identical with how the mind of the subject identifies with the Other, and turns this Other into an identity of the subject through which the subject apprehends the external world.

So as we see, the argument is circular. The law of contradiction is the law of non-contradiction or non-duality, and the law of non-contradiction is the law that by rejecting contradiction cements contradiction and duality.

Just because a singular contradiction may reveal a real truth operative in reality, does not mean that all contradictions are true. If you say that it is day time, now in a particular time zone, it is not also true that it is night time in the same time zone. On the other hand, if you say that there is darkness in light and light in darkness, then this is a statement on an enterily different logical level.

For example, Saturnalia or the dark sun of high noon, refers to how depressed people may feel the most depressed during the time of the day when the sun is at its peak or closest to the earth. They feel depressed or dark inside and they stay inside with shades close shut.

On the other hand, when someone is manically happy, then at midnight they may precisely be at their peak of alertness and activity and be very disturbing to their loved ones or neighbors. The world in mood disorders is upside down precisely because upside down are relative concepts relative to the parameters by which you measure up and down.

The ceiling is up in the north pole but it is down in the south pole from the perspective of the north pole and the same is true vice versa.

We say that the sun sets and the sun rises, but these statements are relative to place and the vantage point of observation. The sun itself neither rises nor sets but simply burns, orbits, turns, and shines bright. The illusion of light and dark is given by the motion of the earth relative to the sun. Then at some point a star may implode as a result of the pull of its own gravity and become a dark sun or black hole that has light but the light cannot escape the intense gravitational pull and therefore cannot be observed.

The different types of logic seem to reflect the body-mind dualism between the physical and the mental. Perhaps it would be safe to assume that true contradictions only appear at a mental level or a level of self reference or mind reference that only applies to the study of human beings. The principle that accepts contradictions or finds them meaningful is a necessary logical principle to understand the human mind itself rather than simply using the human mind to understand nature.

For example, the statement attributed to Groucho Marx that he would not join a club that accepted him as a member. If he tries to join he is rejected and if he is accepted he rejects them. This only makes sense as a mental phenomenon. People want to join clubs to increase their worth which means that they are not worthy enough otherwise, but if they are accepted then it means that their unworthiness is reflected in the status of the club that accepted them and therefore the club is beneath their aspirations of who they want to be.

Another example of paradox or contradiction within the human mind or mental phenomena and speech would be the liar paradox. This statement is false, or I am lying. If it is false it is true and if it true it is false. If I say I am lying I am saying the truth and if I am saying the truth I am lying.

The only exception I can think of to the principle that true contradictions only apply to the study of the human mind, can be found in quantum theory. In Schrodinger's thought experiment the cat is both alive and dead, and at the sub-atomic quantum level a particle is both particle and wave, or a wave is in all places at the same time regardless of distance (superposition).

In addition, if you say that the principle of contradiction is the name for the function that excludes contradictions from a logical system, then this operation does in fact or by fiat establish another system composed of contradictory elements which in themselves may or may not constitute another parallel world system. There is the world of waking life, where a man is a man and a woman is a woman, and then there is the unconscious world of dreams where a male may be a woman, and a female a man.

In the first case man and woman are physical properties, while in the second they are psychical properties (a woman is a female but wants to be a man so in the dream she is represented as a man). Mind has the capacity to formulate true contradictions, while the body seems to be ruled by binary or dual non-contradictions (although not absolutely since there are some cases of hermaphroditism). With the body, the body/brain is either sleeping or awake, but the mind can be asleep while awake, or awake while it sleeps. A body produces a mind, that is not identical with it, and the mind produces a dream body that is not identical with the physical body of the dreamer.

If we take contradictions not as random phenomena, that only appear random because we don't understand them (according to the dialectical function of reason), but consider contradictions as constituting necessary information to understand reality, then contradictions and paradox can be used to include the truth value of a proposition into a larger structure of truth values as I have done above. In such cases, then we do in fact have two parallel logical and rational systems that themselves can either be opposed to each other or overincluded into a larger structure.

Matte-Blanco (1975) uses the terms symmetrical and asymmetrical instead of contradiction and non-contradiction to describe different logical modalities although he only considers formal or binary logic as logic proper, probably under the influence of Bertrand Russell and analytical philosophy and in disregard of continental thought.

He gives the example of the propositional function applied to the relation between a father or a son, or a mother and daughter. The function for the relations between terms/subjects is father of or mother of. In the logic of non-contradiction, that Rene is the father of Raul contradicts the opposite proposition that Raul is the father of Rene. The first is true and the second false. For analysis or for analytical purposes (ironically the word analysis here is used differently than how is used to describe analytical philosophy), there are mental ways in which Raul may be the father of Rene, or play the role of Rene's father, but strictly speaking in the physical/material world and its rules, the father function can only be instantiated once: Rene is Raul's father.

The traditional authority relationship is assymetrical, while the egalitarian approach to authority is symmetrical. In the case of psychoanalysis, for example, Ferenzci's intent to make the analyst-analysand a mutual or symmetrical relationship failed because even if both parties are analysts only one of them is occupying the analytical function. This is true despite the fact that this function precisely also includes the knowledge of symmetrical, non-contradictory, and non-dual phenomena at work in the mind. When asymmetry includes rather than rejects symmetry (as well as vice versa), then asymmetrical logic is a higher level logic than symmetry, since symmetry does not include asymmetry.

When asymmetry rejects symmetry and vice versa, then the rivalry between the systems is on and they both mutually exclude each other. The social sciences according to the model of measurement and computation prevalent in the United States, are an example of the asymmetry that rejects symmetry, while the natural sciences, once the asymmetrical principle is established, can remain open to the humanities and to the principle that includes contradictions, while the humanities remain open to the asymmetrical principle that makes a generative use of the symmetries found in the social-mental worlds.

For Matte-Blanco the symmetrical unconscious represents a modal form of the unrepressed unconscious but this only applies to the unrepressed Id. The unconscious censor that unconsciously represses without being repressed is not symmetrical since it involves the unconscious operation of the function of Sense that necessarily involves establishing difference and classes among things. The primary process can be used for purposes of the drive or for purposes of censorship.

I have shown how a function or the Sense function can function in language and numbers. In language a function can work as sense or meaning, the latter includes censorship as a Code (i.e., erase particular words/values from speech or writing), and can also be used to construct sentences and propositions. Sense or function can also be mathematical or arithmetical and refer to functions within numbers (i.e., multiplication of a number by itself).

But beyond arithmetical operations, can numbers or symbols themselves be used as Code rather than simply as variables or components of the function? In other words, if numbers are not the code but the argument, is there a code for numbers and can the arguments be something else other than numbers and letters?

We have numbers as input but the output can be another number or the geometric form of a biological organism or the physical levels and forms of matter. An example would be the numeric amplitude of a sound wave and how it is perceived as either a pleasant musical sound or a painful signal of distress. There is the number at work in the sound wave that determines its size and form, and then there is the experience of sound as pleasing or harsh. The number is the input/object/reference, the wave is the sense used (hearing), and the pleasant or unpleasant sound is the conscious or mental experience of the sound in a subject.

All of this taken together is the Code, that for the most part is unconscious but not repressed. The only exclusively biological element is the sense modality. But the sense modality will not work without the cultural codes embedded in perception. There may in fact be a harmonious combination or a golden ratio at work in the creation/construction of the universe which is also used by humans to construct a human cultural and mental environment.

Thus, the question can be raised whether there can be hidden connections not only between particular variables but also between the various codes at work in nature. The objects or inputs/outputs for the function may vary, although the function always transforms one into the other for various purposes associated with the various functions.

In this sense, the Code is not necessarily a mental phenomenon or phenomena of Mind and culture (Sense). But since science is first a product of culture more than nature, then it can be argued that cultural Law is the incomplete function that allows for different functions to be substituted in the place of the Code function [( ) ( )]. A function may be the S( ) function and the inputs or variables vary accordingly, or the function itself may vary although it always relates two sets of terms. The first bracket is the placeholder void/place for the various Sense functions while the second void is the empty place for the various arguments.

In the case of numbers both the function and the argument can be made of numbers. Within the code provided by numbers there are prime numbers that function as the building blocks of the code, or the code of the code, so to speak. Prime numbers are the indivisible elements/particles that can only be divided by themselves or 1. Any other number can be made by combining primes, and if any prime numbers are missing then there will also be other numbers absent from a series. Thus, in the case of prime numbers and whole numbers, prime numbers would be the Code or Sense, and natural numbers or integers would be the arguments.

Numbers are written into the very symmetry of the structure inside our bodies and the forms of organisms and the modes of reproduction that secure the survival of the individual and the species. The Code in this case could be Pi in its relations to the various numbers embedded in the geometric forms of nature (rocks and coastlines, microorganisms and organs, for example).

Fractals as apparently random geometric figures found in nature would be another example of a geometric code within mathematics. Each form or shape follows the self-similar logic that each part of the structure has the same property as the whole. The pattern repeats itself according to the imperative to grow and further divide or branch out. Numbers also dictate the arrangement or structure of atoms and subatomic particles.

The mathematically modelled Symbolic order, consists of the triad of Sense or mental function, the arguments or the input/output of words/numbers and senses, and the sense objects that are apprehended by the structure as output. This is the what of the structure and how the structure appears in the imaginary totality of visual perception.

The meaning derived from imaginary totality and shape can then distract us from our desire to know the truth, in the sense of the emergence of the impossible, that is, the unnamable within the Symbolic, that emerges as a structure that lies hidden or does not exist from the view of the Imaginary or the semblance of visual perception. From the perspective of the Imaginary, the underlying mathematical structure both is and is not.

Natural numbers appear to be ordered by logical or rational succession but in fact may be ordered by a ratio of irrational numbers such as the golden number or Pi that continue to infinity. Mathematical structure does not exist in how numbers appear. You have to actually measure the shapes of nature and carry out arithmetical operations in order for the underlying so-called irrational ratio to appear.

In psychoanalysis we don't perform arithmetical operations to reveal the irrational within the structure, but rather use the rules of substitution and metaphor to arrive at the 'what' of the underlying structure that appears not to exist within the phenomenal or manifest figures of speech and discourse. In addition, the structure can also be said not to exist in that structure is not the same as its instantiation in the phenomenal world, and is not the same as the impossible and unnamable that is actually what we are seeking for in the search for truth and knowledge.

The different forms of reason correspond to the different logical levels. There is the cognitive function (understanding) associated with the measurement of forms, and then there is the cogito (dialectical/critical reason or reason proper) linked to the apperception of structure that itself requires Nous (negative dialectics and non-knowing) to apprehend its emptiness and non-existence as the impossible and unnamable or unknowable at work in the emergence of structure and creation.

Practical reason or ethics here has the function of preventing the confusion or collapsing/reducing the different logical levels and dimensions of reality. I would argue that it is not ethical or in the best interest of humanity to define knowledge in the absence of one or more dimensions of rationality.

Conflicts emerge between the different forms of reason, and the discourses they are embedded in, resulting in petty bickering and academic posturing and domination and the fight over economic resources that is rampant in the master's discourse that runs and prevails within university discourse. We have to have the courage to embrace the four forms of rationality that Aristotle and the Greeks have bequeathed us.

Finally, the non-existence of structure is revealed in negative and imaginary numbers (In the case of imaginary numbers or i, the Sense function is the square root of –1). These numbers show that numbers don't have to make sense in the physical world or even in arithmetic (in the case of imaginary numbers). If being childless represents a –1, in the x axis of positive and negative numbers, having a child does not add up to 1 but to 0 (–1 + 1 = 0) which makes sense in mathematics but not in the real world (Romanowicz, 2016).

The square root of −1 does not exist arithmetically or as a number (a negative number multiplied by itself yields a positive number) and yet it can be made to function within arithmetical systems. A structure composed of imaginary numbers does not exist and yet such abstract non-existence can have real practical application. Although imaginary numbers don't exist, they have real practical applications. For air space control at airports, for example, a radar uses the pulse of radio waves to give the position of aircraft in terms of speed and direction. Calculations with imaginary numbers yield the pattern of how radio waves interact.

If we asked which is the ultimate interpretant code, the competition would be on. Whether physical forces, the genetic code or DNA, a mathematical system of numbers, the mental NoF that generates the function of substitution and metaphor in language, or something more akin to habit in the pragmatic orientation, they would all be candidates to occupy the place of being the ultimate interpretant Code.

For Peirce, the signifier/representation represents the object for another signifier-signified (representamen/interpretant) that functions as an interpretant. Would this be another way of saying that the signifier represents the object for someone or a person not defined as another signifier? This of course would differ from Lacan's (S11, p. 207) formula: the signifier is what represents a subject for another signifier given that the someone or the ego of the person cannot escape determination by the signifier and neither can the object. However, the subject typically does not think of itself as a signifier, and yet the subject occupies the place of the signifier.

In this sense it would be more accurate to say that the signifier is what represents an object for another signifier. So are object and subject here occupying the same place in relation to the signifying system? Not quite because we cannot have an object or a signifier without a subject.

Thus, Lacan's formula is more fundamental. But what would stop us from accurately saying that the signifier is what represents an object for a subject or someone as Lacan defines the sign? The problem, of course, is that the subject is another signifier.

From a descriptive or phenomenological formulation, that the signifier represents an object to a subject, may make the most sense to people. Everyone can assume that 'someone' refers to the person or what they think or feel about who they are or what a person or someone should be (please see the upcoming chapter on this topic). However, what the individual thinks, wishes or fantasizes in the Imaginary, is not necessarily what the subject is at a structural level.

Thus Lacan replaces the object and the concept of someone within the formula for the signifier: the signifier is what represents a subject for another signifier. To interpret this formula we must bear in mind that in Lacanian theory signifiers and subjects are interchangeable terms: the subject is what represents the signifier for another subject. The signifier represents Sense and the subject is the reference.

But for the behavioral point of view, the subject is not an objective signifier, but the place of idiosyncratic subjectivism. The final interpretant for Peirce and pragmatism is a habit rather than a Code or the NoF.

Behavioral habits can be thought in various ways. Habitual behaviors can be performed unconsciously/unself-consciously and mechanically. By the way these two are not the same. Learning can be by joyless rote or by the jouissance of meaning and heart, by memory or intelligence. Unconsciously and mechanically in dull habit, is not the same as unconsciously or without self-consciousness, spontaneously, creatively as in music or the aesthetic experience. Mechanically, also indicates a division within the subject between body and mind, while mindfulness is not the same as self-consciousness or even awareness. Does the lack of self-consciousness indicate that something is unconscious or rather points to a form of awareness without self-consciousness? How can awareness and the unconscious arise together, or is'nt this a contradiction in terms? Awareness of ego-consciousness is not the same as awareness of the unconscious.

When I speak about the unconscious in this context what I mean is the unconscious in a descriptive sense that remains capable of consciousness rather than the repressed unconscious. Awareness is what witnesses the flow of the unconscious and unconscious activity but without self-consciousness. The only difference is whether the so-called active flow of mentation is experienced, as a compulsion in the here and now (conscious but without pliable awareness), or as enlightened practice in the step-by-step/moment-by-moment embodiment of reason and structure in human activity.

The Ucs.Pcs. is the storehouse of tacit knowledge or know-how that works automatically, machine like, unconsciously in a descriptive sense but not without awareness. Periodically tacit knowledge, habit, or basic assumptions, need to be questioned in order to make adjustments and acquire new knowledge that will actualize or improve the beauty, truth-value, and efficiency of human action. Efficiency here relies not only on what is said in narrative statements but what remains unsaid and unread in the contextual background of a structure.

This is what is different between how linguistics and psychoanalysis conceive of the message between addresser/sender and addressee/receiver. The message in linguistics is simply the statement or the said, while the saying and the enunciation refer to the subject/signifier of the unconscious whether in analysis or everyday conversation. This dimension of speech is not accounted for in linguistics other than as a form of connotation but connotation opens up to conceptual interpretations that are not the same as a fresh, spontaneous utterance from the unconscious.

We have to be able to trust the storehouse unconscious (in a descriptive sense) that provides parameters for experience and perception and for trust in the reality of perception and the external world. Tacit understandings and supporting assumptions generate a sense of ontological security or what Winnicott would call a going-on-being.

It is interesting to observe the difference between a trust in tacit knowledge and memory, that implies an acceptance of the benevolence of the symbolic/parental order, and the trust in the mother's desire and care giving that for the child functions as a background for independent activity in the world.

Both forms of trust appear to be predicated on the paternal/parental metaphor, the trustworthiness of the word and of the mother's desire. The heteronomy of the Other and the unconscious is accepted as a source of creativity rather than rejected as interfering with ego autonomy.

However, in contrast to Winnicott, or ideas of secure attachment to the mother, Freud believed that tacit knowledge may induce a false sense of security in a false construction of the world. The world is believed to be what is perceived and yet the tacit knowledge leading to perception may provide false knowledge regarding the world however much this false knowledge may serve as a basis for a shared consensual reality.

In this sense, true doubt, the suspension of assumptions, and an unassuming attitude may be as important as trust and faith in the Other of tacit knowledge. The desire of the mother may be a supportive assumption to make and yet may be equally experienced as an engulfing or anxiety producing presence. The same can be said about the NoF, it can be experienced as a trust in the word and the symbolic order, or as a negating or negative influence on the subject.

In addition, the automatism of habit is used in good and bad habits. Habits can be healthy or unhealthy, good or bad, vice or virtue. On the other hand, when habits are performed as a practice of awareness then they are no longer performed mechanically and habit is deautomatised. To avoid mindless routines or habitual mechanical behavior, habit has to function within mind consciousness and not simply be programmed by a binary computer or positive reinforcement.

Paradoxically a robot, puppet, or a wooden subject, may function efficiently due to the absence of personal will or resistance, or a robotic performance could indicate something routinary and habitual performed by rote according to plan and program but without the creative and fresh spontaneity or aliveness of the psyche. The function performed by a robot may provide a semblance of fresh and spontaneous efficiency but the robot cannot function without the human programmer. The Other of the unconscious instead is organically integrated into the function of the human subject.

According to the faculty of sense, and the organ of sight, the object is an icon read as a trace or mark that represents a proximity not only to the presence but also more importantly to the absence of the object.

Thus trace may be a better term than index, which is the sign used by Peirce to represent proximity to the object, because proximity can be proximity to the presence or absence of the object. The unary trace is a better term than index because the unary trace as the mark of the unmarked includes both presence and absence. In Seminar XI Lacan calls the *objet a* the index of a void.

In this formulation 'firstness' instead of the object, represents the unary trace, the mark of the unmarked, and the loss of the object or S_0.

'Secondness' refers to the S_1 or the signifier and the substance of expression.

Thirdness is S_2 or the Code.

The concept represents the object for another interpretant (habit). A habit for Pierce is an ultimate interpretant because it does not change and gets repeated over and over again. But the same could be said of any Code.

According to Lacan the signifier (representamen) is what represents the subject for another signifier/signified/interpretant. The signifier is not what represents something (an object) to someone (the definition that Lacan [1964] gives of the sign). Someone here is a habit (character) in the case of Peirce and another signifier in the case of Lacan.

Habit as an interpretant can be the representation of a drive, an inborn or inherent impulse/disposition for action that is also affected by the action itself either by selecting and reinforcing or inhibiting and not using or extinguishing the dispositions.

Ontogeny and individual development refer to acquired characteristics/dispositions, but phylogeny refers to evolution and inborn physiological dispositions of the organism that are passed on through sexual reproduction. However, in human sexuality there is so much more than reproduction and from this follows the question whether the fantasized, imaginary, and symbolic dimensions of human sexuality are an acquired or an inborn characteristic. The capacity to imagine, to represent, and to speak, is genetic or inborn, but the content and the structure within which the capacity operates is acquired.

References

Frege, G. (1892 [1992]). *Meaning and Reference* (A. W. Moore, Ed.). New York: Oxford University Press.

Freud, S. (1933). *New Introductory Lectures on Psycho-Analysis*. SE, 22, 3–182.

Kristeva, J. (1941 [1980]). *Desire in Language*. New York: Columbia University Press.

Lacan, J. (1964 [1981]). *The Four Fundamental Concepts of Psychoanalysis*. New York: Norton.

Lacan, J. (1975–1976 [2016]). *The Seminar of Jacques Lacan, Book XXIII*, J. A. Miller (Ed.). Cambridge: Polity Press.

Matte-Blanco, I. (1975). *The Unconscious as Infinite Sets. An Essay in Bi-logic*. London: Karnac.

Moncayo, R. (2017). *Lalangue, Sinthome, Jouissance, and Nomination. A Reading Companion and Commentary on Lacan's Seminar XXIII on the Sinthome*. London: Karnac.

Muller, J. P. (1996). *Beyond the Psychoanalytic Dyad. Developmental Semiotics in Freud, Pierce, and Lacan*. New York: Routledge.

Peirce, C. S. (1867 [2009]). *The Essential Peirce: Selected Philosophical Writings. Volumes 1 and 2* (Peirce Edition Project, Ed.). Bloomington & Indianapolis: Indiana University.

Peirce, C. S. (1940 [1955]). *Philosophical Writings of Pearce* (J. Buchler, Ed.). New York: Dover.

Romanowicz, M. (2016). A personal conversation.

von Uexküll, T. (1987). The Sign Theory of Jakob von Uexküll. In Krampen et al. (Eds.), *Classics of Semiotics* (pp. 147–179). New York: Plenum.

5

The Ego, the Person, the Self, and the Subject

In response to Lacan's emphasis on Freud's Metapsychology, many have argued that without the second theory of Mind, or what Freud (1923) calls the structural model, Freud would not have had a theory of personality.

In this regard, I would like to pose the question whether Freud needed to construct a theoretical fiction, to account for processes that occur without self, under the pressure of a social ideal of individualism that begun in Europe with the Italian Renaissance.

Building on the topographical model, Lacan wants to account for defenses, the preconscious, and the reality principle by relying on language rather than on the fiction of an autonomous ego or an ego drive for self-preservation. Instead of the illusion of an agent or a master that develops and commands cultural principles, in Lacanian theory the subject is determined by the symbolic order and at the same time there is a dimension of the subject that is not determined by language and remains undetermined within the dimension of the Real.

R. Moncayo, *Knowing, Not-Knowing, and Jouissance*, The Palgrave Lacan Series,
https://doi.org/10.1007/978-3-319-94003-8_5

Personality as a Subset of Mind

Let's start first by defining Mind as distinct from the ego although personality theory is also understood as a branch of psychology or of the theory of Mind. It is important to stress that Freud had a theory of Mind, because otherwise the ego and the personality could simply be understood in behavioral terms as conditioned behavior or as an aggregate of stimulus and response packets under the heading of habits.

Mind implies subjectivity as well as consciousness and its double: The Un-conscious or Ucs. Consciousness is a mental state but what about the Unconscious? All the formations of the Unconscious are mental formations that manifest as mental states as observed in parapraxes, mental states with decreased consciousness (dreams), or mental states of confusion and agitation (anxiety) associated with mental suffering that people often describe as more painful than physical suffering.

The ego is a mental state associated with ego-representations and identifications, and with narcissistic libido. The ego is not the same as consciousness, since for Freud the ego also extended into the Unconscious in the form of unconscious defenses. From this it follows that the ego can represent unconscious states of mind. The ego can be identified with bodily processes, narcissistic identifications, and defenses. The ego appropriates things that are without self or ego: physical processes, thing or imaginary representations, and verbal or linguistic representations.

Along the way, it is important to underscore that Freud did have a theory of consciousness despite his focus and discovery of the concept of the repressed Unconscious. As presented in the first chapter, his theory of consciousness is also not the same as the concept of ego representations because consciousness in the latter case is associated with the registration of objects in the preconscious system. Consciousness in the preconscious system is associated with an object of consciousness that is apprehended within a representational linguistic system. This is the Pcs.Cs. system rather than the Pcpt.Cs. system.

Perception divides into Pcpt.Cs. and Pcs.Pcpt.Cs. The former is a quality of Cs. that does not retain mnemic traces, while the latter does.

In the case of preconscious perception consciousness arises together with the object that is apprehended according to the levels of the sign and mental structure, and the different dimensions of experience.

Thus, as argued in Chapter 1, consciousness in the Pcpt.Cs. system is a form of empty awareness that receives new impressions without retaining traces and this differs from consciousness of an object in the Pcs.Cs. system. However, even though perception in the Pcs.Cs., associated with becoming aware, involves thinking and language, ego and object representations, pure perceptive awareness of the senses, solely involves intellective capacities and functions. At this level of experience, the intellect is involved in appraising forms and identifying the objects of the various senses and their distinctions: hearing, seeing, etc. Such perception takes place unconsciously in the sense of the descriptive unconscious or despite where the objects of consciousness may be at the time. While perception of the external world takes place, consciousness may be day dreaming about Pcs. associations that may be linked to repressed unconscious contents.

Pure perception involves a form of thinking/cognition that does not involve ego-representations or conscious deliberation at all. Awareness of the world is a function of the clear state that does not retain impressions as well as the registrations that have been laid down in the Pcs. without the latter saturating awareness or the Pcs. system with ego representations. From this vantage point it is possible to think of the Pcs. Cs. system and the ego as two different although potentially related concepts. They are not two names for the same thing but rather two different names for different concepts and phenomena.

Freud identifies the conscious part of the ego with the seat of reason. However, there is more than one type of reason, and this is something that Freud did not consider at least in a systematic way. The aspect of the ego that functions according to ego-representations, narcissistic investments, and aggressiveness, conflicts with the impartiality associated with reason in science. But the awareness and pure intellect associated with preconscious perception of the external world would in fact be consistent with the principles of science.

Freud's use of categories derived from philosophy and the history of ideas (*vorstellung*-representations, for example) differs from how the concept of representation is used nowadays in cognitive science, whether cognitive behaviorism or computational theories of mind. The latter follows the belief that science can disregard the history of ideas or philosophy in favor of a current and narrow formal definition of rationality. This is also the difference between an intellectual and a scientist, although nowadays scientists are considered intellectuals except for the fact that the natural scientist operates with a restricted notion of rationality divorced from intellectual history and philosophy.

Neither of these things is true in Freud or psychoanalysis except that his theory of the ego does seem to fit this model. The theory of cognition associated with the ego and the function of reality testing appears to reflect Descartes modern theory of the cogito: "I think therefore I am." However, Freud said that the ego is not the master in his/her own house, but this refers to the Id and the drives and not to the unconscious cognition reflected in Lacan's (1966–1967) permutation of the Cartesian cogito: from "I think, therefore I am" to "I think where I am not" (Session 5: Wednesday 14 December 1966).

Analytical philosophy or the philosophy of science that supports technical procedures, formal reason, and techne, neglects nous, dialectical logic, and practical reason. Psychoanalysis uses the four Aristotelian categories of reason and this is what lends it a broad, profound, and humane dimension derived from a founding genius. I say genius because most of the geniuses that the history of the university depends on were only post facto incorporated and accepted into academic discourse.

There are many examples: Socrates, Newton, Darwin, Einstein, Freud and Lacan, to name only a few. Profound theoretical creativity often occurs outside the university. In the social sciences, empiricist (statistical) science operates according to rational models based on formal analytical reason and techne. The latter are shared with binary digital computers and with artificial intelligence but may lack a properly human dimension.

Practical reason is so much more than technical rationality. Praxis not only includes ethics, but also a practice of the Real or a Real practice that involves subjectivity, or an objective form of subjectivity independent from quantitative measurement. The practice of the Real incorporates the timeless, non-categorical dimension of the unconscious that is either beyond language or that uses a different modality of language.

Nous in turn represents non-knowing rather than the not-knowing associated with ignorance. This non-knowing is linked to the repressed unconscious, the Real unconscious, the position and listening of the analyst, and the clear state that does not retain impressions. To change the relation that a thought/representation has to a form of jouissance/experience, one has to not-know the belief associated to the representation. Not-knowing or ignorance can mean "I do not-know the cognitive bias or false beliefs that operate in perception," or "I know the distortions and chose to ignore them," or "I make corrections and introduce changes to the emotional response to beliefs, and hold beliefs with more dispassion, equanimity, and flexibility." This form of disbelief or creative doubt linked to science, allows for jouissance to be re-linked to repressed or new representations/signifiers.

A practice of the Real is exemplified by analytical practice but is not limited to the acts of a psychoanalyst. Meditation, Yoga and related body-arts, Theatre, Experiment, Writing, Visual arts, are all practicing the praxis of the Real. In all these practices, one can differentiate among content, form, and emptiness or void/lack. The goal is in the activity/practice itself. They are all forms of human activity but also examples of enlightened activity. When human activity is defined solely by habit or repetitive actions without access to the Real, circling endlessly between the Symbolic and the Imaginary, then we have praxis in the sense of human activity but no enlightened activity.

On the other hand, it is difficult to separate enlightened activity from ordinary habitual activity because enlightenment cannot be reified. To separate the two would be to reify enlightenment, but to not differentiate habitual activity from enlightened activity is to ignore the Real and ignoring how to even begin to recognize what in experience is unknown or even unknowable.

A letter of emptiness, or a Real gesture, a sound, a sudden illumination, the beginning or the end of something, the act as an event in the present moment, is what places a mark on the infinite line that appears thanks to the mark. This is the Real unconscious that resists or places an obstacle on symbolization, specially standardized symbolization.

Listening is also a Real practice facilitated by the clear state acting as a screen/filter to prevent past experience from saturating and biasing new and present experience. One listens with knowing, not-knowing or ignoring, and non-knowing that allows for the emergence of new significations.

Finally, the episteme that links theory and practice include dialectical reason/logic and contradiction, and not simply formal logic and the principle of non-contradiction. The mind as construed by Freud includes many antithetical or contradictory phenomena, as seen in dreams, the antithetical meaning of primal words, the formations of the unconscious, symptoms, the experience of pain and pleasure, and the reversible quality of the pleasure and reality principle, of primary and secondary process thinking and feeling states (love and hate for example). Formal reason and techne alone, although rational, cannot capture the observations of psychoanalysis and the dimensions of human subjectivity it studies.

Coming back to the ego, I have argued that the ego differs from consciousness insofar as the ego is the agent of defense. The ego avoids unpleasure and in its attempts to bind the energy of repressed representations, the repressive efforts become contaminated by the repetition compulsion associated with the primary process. But in this explanation the ego would not be unconscious. Rather the unconscious primary process would absorb ego processes.

In addition, in the Ego and the Id Freud describes the Pcpt.Cs. system as living neuronal tissue that adapts to the external world and is differentiated out of the Id. On the other hand, the ego is the product of identifications and is made up of representational elements. The ego is both the person and an agency or instance within the psyche. The ego is also the object of narcissistic libido and the site of self-love, self-respect, and pride. In addition, the ego is supposed to represent a principle of union and synthesis as it struggles to reconcile the opposing tendencies of reason or Law and passion. Both latter tendencies consist of representations or ideals and repression takes place when the dominant mass of ideas that represent the ego are in conflict or oppose/reject the ideas that will be repressed.

An alternative explanation is to consider the principle of enverity as articulated by Bristow (2017). The ego does not mediate; rather it is the subject that finds itself on one side or another of the Moebius strip. On the Moebius strip, sometimes the subject finds itself on the side of consciousness and sometimes on the side of the unconscious. The unconscious side of the Moebius strip coincides with the enunciating subject while the conscious side represents the ego of the statement. The ego represents the unified persona of the one or two-dimensional social individual that is mostly imaginary from a Lacanian point of view.

To incorporate the two sides of the Moebius strip requires a three-dimensional bubble that would include the back of the subject and the blind spots in the field of vision where the gaze of the Other sees the subject. "I know you are looking but I will pretend I don't know, but don't let me catch you." From a special place of *aphanisis* or the vanishing point, "I see you seeing me." Sense perception surrounds all beings like a bubble. As I see, I know I am equally being seen but is there a difference in this seeing? Who is seeing? If there is no one there and only seeing is seeing, then couldn't we change the observer without affecting the experience? Logically it makes sense, except that everyone's subjective experience of the external environment is different.

Lacan starts out from the early Freud (1893–1895) and the discovery of a *Spaltung* or division in the psyche (a splitting or dissociation in consciousness) as revealed in the clinical examples of neurosis. At first this division in the personality appeared to be purely pathological particularly in contrast to the unified 'persona' of the social individual. However, such mask or persona turns out to be purely imaginary. There is no boundary between normality and neurosis, only a difference between neurosis with symptoms and neurosis or character neurosis without symptoms. In so-called normal character, the symptoms are the distinguishing traits of the personality and the jouissance contained therein.

The ego remains symptomatic despite the unary trait or because of it. The symptomatic aspect of an ego trait reveals the division of the subject. The ego feels at one with the trait as part of who they are, but who they are in the sense of the trait, puts them at odds with the Other.

What Freud transposes from pathology to normality is that the division of the subject in hysteria or neurosis reveals the actual structure of the psyche. The psyche or mind is composed of two or three, or even four levels. The ego grapples with the super ego and the Id and is itself an aggregate or composite of these elements.

With the second theory, Freud personalizes what in the first theory of mind were structural symbolic effects. Lacan emphasizes that defenses take place within language and within the functions of metaphor and metonymy as described by Jakobson (1990). A metaphor substitutes for something else in the same way that a symptom does, except that in the symptom there is a quantum of jouissance (conflicting affects) that is displaced unto the substitute. We say yes when we intend to say no or vice versa. There is a metonymical displacement from no to yes as well as a metaphoric substitution. At the same time, there is a change in sign in the quanta from positive to negative, from pleasure to pain. Pleasure and pain are not symmetrical since pleasure can be experienced in both increases and decreases of tension while pain is only experienced with an increase in tension or pressure.

Metaphors and ideals guide and censor (the direction of sense) thought rather than the ego being the source of censorship. In Freud's second theory it is unclear whether the unconscious ego is the super ego or whether the super ego and ego both have conscious and unconscious dimensions. If the latter is the case, then what is the difference between the unconscious ego and the unconscious super ego in terms of the function of unconscious defense? This in fact is difficult if not impossible to ascertain and it points to a dead end in the second theory of mind and personality.

The repressions of the ego are carried out on behalf of the ego ideal and the super ego that state 'do this' and 'don't do that'. When the ego can identify the ego ideal and the super ego as his/her own, then the ideals are syntonic rather than ego dystonic. Freud attributes to the early real ego the inhibitory function involved in the inhibition of early hallucinatory wish fulfillment that takes place in a small infant. The reality ego focuses on utility and preventing damages. Hallucinatory wish-fulfillment is not effective and threatens to damage the relation to the real breast.

But how can the ego repress before there are any ego representations or a repressive ego? According to Freud, what allows the ego to repress is a stable quantity/quality of energy also known as bound or quiescent energy. This is how object relations, ego psychology, and self-psychology define the self: a sense of calm trust, a secure attachment, a feeling of being loved by the Other, and a belief in the world as a benevolent place represented by the symbolic mother and father. But again, such reservoir of stable potential or kinetic energy exists before the ego and constitutes the energetic origins of the ego or is the ego the one that initiates the secondary process? Freud says that the real ego exists before the pleasure ego and before the reality principle is established.

Perhaps we just like to use the name ego to designate stable energy or the function of metaphor. There is a rudiment of both pleasure and inhibition that could just as well be attributed to inhibitions in the transmission of impulses along a neuronal chain or to the inhibitions imposed by language and symbolization. Perhaps this is what Freud meant by the unconscious ego: the epigenetic transmission of the superego from one generation to the next as a pattern or types of inhibitory mechanisms of nerve cells.

With the invention of narcissistic libido, Freud (1914) describes how object cathexes and investments are incorporated into the ego through identifications. Does identification desexualize object libido when transformed into narcissistic libido or does the ego operate with the non-sexual energy of the drive for self-preservation? Structurally, absolute primary narcissism precedes the distinction between subject and object rather than being an abnormal fixation to a primitive stage of development. There is no earlier state of the ego prior to the subject-object distinction. The fixation to the ideal ego does not precede the fixation to the object. The fixation to the object in relative primary narcissism precedes the fixation to the ego since the ego represents identification with the object.

The Ideal Ego

Elsewhere (Moncayo, 2008) I dedicated a chapter to differentiating four degrees within narcissism. In the first level, we find absolute and relative primary narcissism that include a state without a subject or object differentiation, and a narcissism of the object, however paradoxical this may sound; the ideal ego is the second degree of narcissism; the ego ideal is the third. The fourth degree is associated with benevolent depersonalization, subjective destitution and the traversal of the fantasy. While the first three are in Freud, the fourth degree is clearly associated with Lacanian theory and the end of analysis. The fourth degree coincides with what Lacan (1975–1976) calls a new ego in the Real. In addition, following Lacanian theory a clear conceptual distinction can be established between the ideal ego and the ego ideal.

What I mean by narcissism of the object or of a narcissistic object is not what is usually considered to be a characteristic of a narcissistic personality and a fixation to the body image. For Lacanians this latter phenomenon represents a fixation to the ideal ego. The narcissism of the object refers to the object of fantasy even before there was an ego. In hallucinatory wish fulfillment, the fixation is with the *objet a* or the fantasy of the breast. This quality of the object of fantasy is used to describe a neonatal and early, if not primitive, form of mental functioning that continues throughout life as a modality of the imaginary sexual relation to the Other sex.

From the breast as an object cause of desire, to weaning and the separation from the breast, to the acquisition of the body image as a replacement for the mother's gaze and breast, the image in the clear mirror represents the body image of the child as the child's own image but also as the object cause of the mother's desire. The child identifies with the object of the mother's desire, who or what she sees in the child that is not the child's but the mother's.

However, through the specular image the object becomes the child's own Ideal Ego (i[a]). Through the specular image the child acquires a bodily identity and a unified body image. The object of the drive is what transmits the drive to the ideal ego (a → a'). The representations of the drive appear as representations of the object. But what was chaotic, unconscious, and scrambled information about the unconscious object now becomes a unified body image that is two-dimensional. We can't see the back of our heads and yet we know the back is there and that we are three dimensional despite what the mirror says.

Lacan identifies the S (homophony with *Es* [Id or It] in German) of the pre-subject with the It. I argue that in the beginning the non-differentiation between subject and object represents 'It' and in a second moment (relative primary narcissism), the identification with the object breast represents the Id. In this formulation, it is important to remember that in the non-differentiation between subject and object, as seen in the example of intrauterine life, the subject and the object are still connected through the placenta that Lacan considers as one of the first *objet a*.

Absolute primary narcissism is a state where the libido is stored both in the It and in the S or pre-subject. In relative primary narcissism libido emanates from the object but also from the ego since the ego is identified with the object that is the first form of ego. In relationship to the breast, energy is sexualized and when the ego desexualizes object libido it is simply returning to the prior condition where energy emanates both from the pre-subject and the object.

Freud says the ego is a bodily ego which first means an organismic ego and secondly a body image that replaces the primary object. The body image is a two-dimensional surface reflected in a mirror (mother's eyes, water, metal surface, or modern clear mirror). But Freud also says the ideal ego is a mental projection of the surface of the body and a projection of the organism unto the mind. The body becomes the mind in the specular image or the ideal ego.

The ideal ego becomes a long-lasting structure of the subject, more than a pathological fixation that needs to be abandoned. The specular image becomes pathological if the lack in the image is not symbolized in the direction of the ego ideal.

The Ego Ideal

In the previous work mentioned above, following Freud's idea of degrees of differentiation within narcissism, and Lacan's distinctions between the ideal ego and ego ideal, I established a difference between the ideal ego constructed on the model of the relationship with the mother in contrast to the ego ideal that is constructed based on the relationship to the father/Other. The ideal in the ideal ego is a body image, while the ideal in the ego ideal and the relationship to the father represents social and intellectual ideals (values, concepts, identifications). The ego ideal is a symbolic body of signifiers of the Other that the ego appropriates and invests with narcissistic libido with a + and – sign. The super ego represents the – sign of the ego ideal.

As the ego ideal provides new aims for narcissism, the super ego embodies imaginary castration and narcissistic injuries. The ego ideal now will mediate narcissism and self-love, self-respect, and pride. The Other and the ego ideal will love the ego if the ego identifies with social ideals and complies and develops good habits for ordinary living. Bad habits represent a defiance of the Other and a rejection of the symbolic castration and compliance/submission embodied in the ego ideal and good habits. The super ego then will castigate (imaginary castration) the ego for the failure to uphold the ego ideals associated with the father and the Other.

The ego ideal can be identified with the narcissism and imaginary function of the Name of the Father and its prestige. The NoF is the signifier and the imaginary phallus is the signified as the object of the mother's desire. In development and symbolic castration, the child stops being the imaginary phallus of the mother and the imaginary phallus becomes the signified of the signifier of the NoF. The father is supposed to have the imaginary phallus that the mother wants, and its signifier is the NoF.

In this perceived move of the desire of the mother from the child to the father, the child goes from omnipotent fusion to castration/loss/separation. Lacanians speak of symbolic castration because the child loses the place of the imaginary object.

The child will then forward to the father the question of the missing object. What the child gets back from the father to compensate for the loss of the object (mother, *objet a*, imaginary phallus) is the NoF or the signifiers/ideals of the father/Other. The loss of the object is also a loss at the level of the ego. The pre-subject becomes the divided subject and the product of the division is the missing object/signifier. The object will always slide metonymically and thus cannot provide a stable identity for the subject. The NoF is what offers a stable metaphor that can stop the sliding and fracturing of the object.

However, the imaginary identification with the father and the imaginary function of the Name does not offer a stable solution to the ego either. It looks like the imaginary NoF can close the gap in the subject, but the narcissistic shine of the Name is always threatened by lack. The search for fame, stardom, fortune, power, are all associated with the imaginary function/trappings of the NoF. These are all attempts to deny or close the lack in the subject. The NoF must move from the Imaginary to the Symbolic (in the sense of accepting the lack and castration in the father as symbolic rather than a real deficit) and from the Symbolic to the Real. In the move from the Symbolic to the Real, the Name reveals rather than conceals the lack while the void as Real acquires a different significance beyond symbolic lack.

The Ego in the Real

The move of the NoF from the Symbolic to the Real, coincides with a further fourth degree differentiation within the ego, from the ego ideal to the ego in the Real. This is the rock of symbolic castration and the most difficult of narcissistic wounds: the symbolic father and phallus are also found to be lacking, a zero or a nothing. Once the illusions regarding the ideal father and the disillusions regarding the lack and limitations of the father have been cleared in the transference to the analyst, the father remains as an empty symbolic function but still a function, nonetheless.

The task of the analyst is to serve as a support for this function by ultimately being empty of content that could define the identity of the analysand. This is the exact opposite of what people ordinarily think the father function to be. The father function is typically associated with the super ego and the ego ideal, with telling people what to do and what not to do. Subjects, however, have to find out things for themselves and shape their own destinies based on the choices they make with the elements that they are made with. The Other cannot give the subject his or her own Being (Lacan, 1958–1959, p. 138).

It is only with the fourth degree of differentiation within narcissism that the subject can rebirth itself (what Lacan calls *se-parere*) past imaginary ego-identifications. The subject is reborn as a new signifier that appears thanks to the autonomy and dynamic self-creating capacity of the Symbolic.

The Symbolic is autonomous or self-organized because it is capable of dynamic change over long periods of time. In addition, it is autonomous from the subject because it conditions the subject rather than the other way around. On the other hand, the subject is autonomous from the Symbolic because it occupies the place of emptiness or a hole or a lack of closure within the structure. In this regard, the autonomy of the subject and the autonomy of the Symbolic seem to meet at this level. To produce a new signifier for the subject from the place where the Other cannot give the subject his or her own Being (the subject of the Real), the new signifier must emerge from the subject but also from the emptiness of the battery of signifiers or the lack in the Other. The lack in the Other, is the place within the Symbolic that gives access to the Real.

The final Lacan argued that the subject is an "answer of the Real" and not "an answer of the Other" or of the Symbolic. However, the autonomy of the subject is empty or devoid of any inherent meaning. It is only within the Imaginary that the ego imputes to itself the function or agency of generating new meaning. New meaning is generated within the Symbolic itself as a function of the interaction between the emptiness of the Real and of the subject and the dynamic interaction between the elements of an open structure under on-going construction.

In the analytical situation, the analyst functions from the place of suspended authority that represents this lack in the Other to define the identity of the subject. The subject is no longer fooled by the *objet a* that appears to fall off the Other but actually falls off from the place of the subject's own fantasy.

Paradoxically, the agency of the subject is limited to the act of leaving empty the place of ego-agency within the structure and the place of the cause of desire within the subject. On the other hand, the larger agency, the autonomy and activity of the Symbolic could also represent the work of a benevolently depersonalized subject. The illusion is that the ego is the agent that advances and realizes things or symbolic causes but instead it is the Symbolic that advances and realizes the subject.

This is not unlike the work of the poet or the metaphoric subject who makes a non-instrumental use of language for new meanings and words to emerge from the Real as the locus of an essential void within the Symbolic. In the Greek myth of Narcissus, Narcissus drowns in a vain attempt to grab his image reflected in the water. But the story does not end there, because in a second moment, in the place where Narcissus fell, the Narcissus flower appears. The narcissus flower represents the new subject.

The recognition of the emptiness of the Other, that Lacan symbolised in the image of the empty mirror without a fixed ego representation, also coincides with what Kohut (1966) called a cosmic narcissism marked not only by joy but also by a solemn and serene inner confidence. The emptiness of the mirror represents the calm and unperturbed nature of the mirror itself (Other jouissance). The mirror equally accepts, holds, and let's go of any image. What Lacan calls the calculated vacillation of the analyst's neutrality refers to this accepting and holding of the images and signifiers that appear in the mirror, but it also means letting them go, a quality that is classically associated with the analyst's neutrality. When the analyst holds the contents of the mirror, the emptiness of the mirror is still there.

Finally, what I am calling a fourth-degree or end state narcissism is differentiated from first-degree primary narcissism (or the oceanic feeling, as Freud called it), because it includes rather than excludes all the mediations/separations introduced by the paternal function. End state narcissism is not a primordial experience of identity with the mother, because within the Symbolic, identity is necessarily different or metaphoric.

Lacan argues that in the final analysis or in the end of analysis the *objet a* dissolves "owing to its failure, unable, as it is, to sustain itself in approaching the Real" (Lacan, 1971–1972, p. 95). When finally, the object is reached in the Real rather than the Imaginary, the object dissolves for this very reason. The mythical union with the One always produces 1 + a. So how can the object vanish without producing a substitute as we just said happens with respect to the approach to the One? Is it the *a* that dissolves or the image of the body?

In the case of Joyce, Lacan argues that in the new ego the image of the body is not involved. This contrasts with the ego in Freud that was a bodily ego but as a libidinal surface or image. Because we identify with the body image we relate to the other through the assumption of similar images, minds, and selves. Nietzsche (1885–1887) said something similar when he wrote: "The assumption of similar cases presupposes 'similar souls'" (p. 276). Soon these assumptions crystallize into concepts leading to the cognitive ego functions of affirmative judgments of attribution or negation: I am this, and you are not, or I am not that and you are this, or this is inside me and that is outside. However, the similarity of body image, racial features, gender, etc. points to the imaginary fact that the more similarity you find the more difference you generate. The similarity or similitude based on the emptiness of the mirror and of the Other that we all share is something different.

At the end of analysis, the i (in the matheme i[a] for ideal ego) and the I (in matheme I[A] or I[O] for ego ideal) can be detached from the *a* and the A/O respectively. This non-attachment signifies having ideas and ideals without idealization or imaginary identifications, to have a father ideal without an ideal father. The Imaginary is separated from the Real (i/a) and from the Symbolic (I/O), freeing the three registers to be re-articulated under the *sinthome*. The Real becomes the Real of the later Lacan: without the Imaginary of "the thing" and the fantasy of the imaginary phallus, the Imaginary becomes the creative Imagination, and the Symbolic contains the Real or where words hit the Real rather than cover it.

The *Je* and the *Moi*, the Ego and the Subject

The hole or lack in the Other (S[Ø]), is the same as saying that there is a −1 inherent in the set of linguistic signifiers. Structurally this means that in speech there is a −1 or a missing signifier in every statement. Lacan (1960) says that this −1 is unpronounceable, but the operation can be pronounced whenever a proper name is pronounced in a statement. 'The operation is the calculation of signification' as follows in Fig. 5.1.

In the picture, the signifier is represented by −1 and the signified is represented as the square root of −1. When the signifier represents −1 and the signified represents square root of −1, the result of their division is −1. However, there is a double meaning to what the missing thing is. On the one hand, there is a missing signifier represented by −1, on the

$$\frac{\text{S (signifier)}}{\text{s (signified)}} = \text{s (the statement)},$$

$$\text{with S} = (-1)\text{, we find: s} = \sqrt{-1}$$

$$\frac{-1}{\sqrt{-1}} = -1$$

Fig. 5.1 The calculation of signification. Romanowicz and Moncayo (2015)

other hand, there is a signifier with no signified (the signified is not missing it just does not exist although it produces effects in speech).

Since Being is located inside the hole of the Other [Ø], Lacan (1960) asks the question: "But where does this being, who appears in some way missing from the sea of proper names, come from?" (p. 694). The answer comes from the Real: "I am in the place from which the universe is a flaw in the purity of Non-being" (ibid.). Birth and death require an impurity within the pure void or emptiness. Without impurity, nothing happens or Being does not manifest. The place of the I is the place of a flaw in the purity of Non-Being and this place Lacan also calls the place of *Jouissance* (or the place of Life and Death, bodily pleasure and pain). The I and *jouissance* share the lack of a signifier, since the signifier is missing or is continually shifting. This is what Lacan calls the flaw in the purity of Non-being. In the Other, beyond a simple and self-referential name or unary trace, there is a lack of a substantial and stable referential signifier for the subject.

It is interesting that Lacan says that the symbolic phallus is the signifier of *jouissance*, while the question of *jouissance* is 'What am I?' Am I my mother's special object or do I have a symbolic identity that the Name and Word designates, or, furthermore, is this symbolic identity simply a signifier rather than an object of jouissance? Both the missing I or substantial subject and the symbolic phallus are signifiers of *jouissance*, yet *jouissance* is also said to not have a signifier and the signifiers themselves are missing. Since the signifier for the symbolic phallus is missing, more and more jouissance cannot be defined either by the object nor the signifier. The subject becomes a trace of jouissance in the Real that, nonetheless, the subject still must take responsibility for. The I represents the subject/letter (S) of jouissance and the place where the I must take responsibility for jouissance and desire (Lacan 1957/2006).

This traceless trace of jouissance is not only an energetic state but also a state of mind consciousness or of the Pcpt.Cs. system that does not retain impressions or representations of the subject or of the object. With respect to this singular trace all the subject can say or become is "This I am", or "I am this", or "Just this."

Does this correspond with the formula for sublimation that Freud gave in the Ego and the Id: "Where Id was, ego shall be"? No because the ideal ego or ego ideal are no longer objects of social utility or signifiers that close the gap in the subject. In the Lacanian graph of desire, the latter would translate into the upper signifying chain being expressed/concealed through the lower narrative of the ego and social discourses that give a tamed interpretation of the drive.

Lacan's (1959–1960) own formula and permutation of Freud's formula is: "Where It was, I shall become" (this or come to being). Lacan uses It instead of Id. By It he means a different concept of the Id. Instead of a chemical soup, chaos, or a seething cauldron of primitive impulses, the It is the "no-thing" as the nature of the object, jouissance, or *das Ding* in the Real as the subject qua-nothing. The Id instead refers to the 'thing' of the archaic object that framed the first form of ego where no boundaries between ego and object exist. The Id represents a form of malevolent depersonalization, where the impersonal dimension of the drive determines the experience of the subject <u>in</u> the Real.

In the subject <u>of</u> the Real the differences between subjects and signifiers is not lost, although the subject is in the gaps-in-between or outside the signifier, and inside the experience of jouissance. The 'no-thing' of the subject is not the same as the 'nothing' that is one of the *objet a*. The 'nothing' as the *objet a* represents the toxic absence of the object. The 'no-thing' is something different that contains both presence and absence and refers to the mystery of the letter and the Name wherein the I is benevolently depersonalized as a form of jouissance.

In addition, I would argue that the I here is the *Je* rather than the *moi* or ego. The *Je* is the subject of jouissance or the "Just This". In front of the image in the mirror of the Other, the subject or *Je* says: I am It, but it is not me. An analysand was bewildered and mildly disturbed by the growing realization in front of the mirror that, as he aged, he looked more and more like his father. He was concerned because he did not want to lose his sense of individuality and individuation.

By mirror of the Other I mean that a mirror is a product of culture while at the same time the empty mirror holds that which is undefined other than as a form of jouissance or energetic intensity. The specular image or ideal ego is me (*Je*) but I (moi-ego) am not It or I am not the image. The *Je* is not defined by the specular image but rather by the empty mirror and the pure capital signifier. Beyond name, language, culture, body and body image, the question of "Who am I," indicates/ instantiates the place of jouissance.

A subject can also say "My father is me, or his desire is mine, but I am not my father and my desire is not his." My father defines my ego but not the *Je* or the I that remains undeterminate. There is something in me (*Je* or jouissance) that cannot be reduced to my father, but this is not the illusory autonomous ego associated with imaginary identifications. The *Je* of the unconscious is a singular empty place within the structure of the Other beyond the biographical father that represents a new place of permutation and transformation for the structure.

If the *Je* said: "I am my father, but my father is not me", the me in the second clause is granting autonomy to the father rather than the subject. The sign and value of the subject is not clear in the example. Assuming there are things in the ego that the subject values over and above the father, then the place of the lack would be in the Other rather than in the *Je*. This state of affairs is a pure form of alienation of the *Je* and of the son in the father represented by the super ego in Freud's second theory of mind.

If the *Je* says "I am not my father", then this opens the door to the *Je* of the S or a significant pure signifier in the Unconscious of a Real jouissance of both the Id and the It. In accessing the object of the drive beyond the father and the father's prohibition, the ego or the *moi* becomes the Id or the pure demand of the sexual drive or of phallic jouissance.

The *Je* of the signifier instead becomes a new signifier of identity that emerges from the Real of jouissance rather than from the ego or from a known battery of signifiers in the Other. This *Je* as It is not the Id, the super ego/ego ideal, or the ego; nor a simple summation of all three. The *Je* is a unary trace of the Pcpt.-Cs. that does not retain ego representations in the Pcs-Cs system and therefore with the unary trace the signifier can be used both by awareness and the Unconscious without requiring the supposition of an ego supposed to know.

References

Bristow, D. (2017). *Joyce and Lacan: Reading, Writing, and Psychoanalysis*. London: Routledge.

Freud, S. (1893–1895 [1966]). *Studies on Hysteria*. New York: Avon Books.

Freud, S. (1914). *On Narcissism: An Introduction*. SE, 14, 67–102.

Freud, S. (1923). *The Ego and the Id*. SE, 19, 3–66.

Jakobson, R. (1990). *On Language*. Cambridge: Harvard University Press.

Kohut, H. (1966). Forms and Transformations of Narcissism. *Journal of the American Psychoanalytic Organization, 14*, 243–272.

Lacan, J. (1957 [2006]). The Instance of the Letter in the Unconscious. In *Ecrits* (B. Fink, Trans). New York: Norton.

Lacan, J. (1958–1959 [1970]). *El Deseo y su Interpretacion. Seminar VI*, O. Masotta (Ed.). Buenos Aires: Nueva Vision.

Lacan, J. (1959–1960 [1992]). *The Ethics of Psychoanalysis. The Seminar, Book VII* (D. Porter, Trans & J. A. Miller, Ed.). New York: Norton.

Lacan, J. (1960 [2006]). The Subversion of the Subject and the Dialectic of Desire. In *Ecrits* (B. Fink, Trans). New York: Norton.

Lacan, J. (1966–1967). *The Seminar of Jacques Lacan. Book XIV. The Logic of Phantasy* (Cormac Gallagher from Unedited French Manuscripts, Trans). Unpublished. Accessed 13 Dec 2017.

Lacan, J. (1971–1972 [1998]). *Encore. The Seminar of Jacques Lacan, Book XX. On Feminine Sexuality, the Limits of Love and Knowledge*. New York: Norton.

Lacan, J. (1975–1976). *Book XXIII. The Sinthome*. Cambridge: Polity Press.

Moncayo, R. (2008). *Evolving Lacanian Perspectives for Clinical Psychoanalysis. On Narcissism, Sexuation, and Jouissance in Psychoanalysis and Culture*. London: Karnac.

Nietzsche, F. (1885–1887). *The Will to Power*. Random House LLC, 2011.

Romanowicz, M., & Moncayo, R. (2015). Going Beyond Castration in the Graph of Desire. *The Letter (The Irish Journal for Lacanian Psychoanalysis), 58*(Spring), 31–58.

6

The Symbolic in the Early Lacan as a Cybernetic Machine, as Automaton and *Tyché*, and the Question of the Real

It is well known that the early period of Lacan's work included a detour through cybernetics. Lacan did not continue this train of thought that was picked up most notably by Guattari (1979) and Deleuze with their notions of the unconscious as a creative machine (the *machinic* unconscious or "*L'inconscient machinique*"). However, as far as I can tell, their notions of desire and of the mind as a machine did not include a detailed incursion into binary logic and computer programming such as that seen in Lacan's exercises at the end of his text on *The Purloined Letter* found in the *Ecrits*. The relation between letters and numbers is complex. On the one hand, letters are meant to be read while numbers are used to perform arithmetical operations and functions. On the other hand, and as Brahnam (2017, a personal conversation) has pointed out, letters as variables can be used to perform arithmetical operations, and numbers can be read symbolically and metaphorically (think of the number 1 for example, as in the phrase: "you are the 1"). Letters and numbers both have an effect outside meaning or can be senseless units that must be combined to generate meaning within a system.

> Drawing upon the work of Friedrich Kittler, Johnston stresses, quite to the contrary, the absolute "*necessity* of cybernetics to Lacan's theory,"

R. Moncayo, *Knowing, Not-Knowing, and Jouissance*, The Palgrave Lacan Series,
https://doi.org/10.1007/978-3-319-94003-8_6

> underscoring that when Lacan says "the symbolic world is the world of the machine," he is referring to computers (Markovian machines, finite state machines, and Turing machines). (Brahnam, p. 30)

Lacan's formulation of the Symbolic as a formal language, incorporates formal logic, Boolean logic, and the binary logic invented by Leibniz and prevailing in the field of computer programming, cybernetics, and cognitive psychology. Lacan's interest in binary logic responds to the attempt to understand and develop Freud's idea that the unconscious determines the conscious ego. He wanted to figure out how a formal language determines the subject even if it is the "active" subject that engages such a language. Like in all logic and mathematics, problems and equations require repeated practice and exercises. This is precisely what Lacan attempts to do in the "Suite" following the text on *The Purloined Letter*.

Such efforts take Lacan outside the parameters used by Freud to define the unconscious. Even though Freud was well-aware of how the unconscious worked within language (in jokes, dreams, and everyday life), Freud believed that images and not words prevailed in the unconscious. It was Lacan's contribution to give an account of the signifying chain operating within the unconscious. However, in 1955 he had not yet developed the concept of the signifying chain with the aid of the graph of desire or the concept of the Real, in its two periods.

Before I continue, it is important to note that there are two published texts on *The Purloined Letter*. One appears in the *Ecrits* (1956 [2006], and the second in Seminar II (1954–1955). Both texts are from 1955–1956, but the *Ecrits* were published in French in 1966, and Seminar II in 1978. It is the text of the *Ecrits* that has the Suite and the Exercises that immediately concern us here and that are discussed in Brahnam's paper. One of the important merits of Lacan's text is how he links Freud's clinical and phenomenological observation of the Fort-Da game in a child, with an exposition of the Even or Odd (Head or Tails) game as it appeared in *The Purloined Letter*. Both serve as examples of how the symbolic order is the world of the machine. *The Purloined Letter* is a short story or mystery by North-American author Edgar Allen Poe.

As the f(O)rt d(A) example or observation constitutes an empirical/structural moment of psychoanalytic developmental theory, the Even/Odd game represents a foundation for probability theory. The result of the combination amounts to an informal proof of how automaton, as a supposed form of chance, or randomness, represents an actual form of causal determination. The probability of a win or a loss is already determined by the structure and articulation between win and loss, head or tails, + or −. This form of chance or randomness is how the Real first appears to Lacan.

I will first examine the concepts of *Automaton* and *Tyché* as they appear in Seminar XI, before returning to the Fort-Da game and the signifying machine presented in the Exercises. Lacan's final concept of the Real is articulated in Seminar XXIII (see Moncayo, 2017).

Tyché and *Automaton*

The early Real is ominous, painful, awful, hazardous, accidental, and is often not differentiated from the concept of reality in general or the two are used interchangeably. The second Real is more like *Tyché*, a true hole that generates consonance and concord, or is benevolent and auspicious. This view coincides with *Tyché* as the Greek goddess of Fortune as something surprising and undetermined at the heart of the structure of determination, the point where structure vanishes or does not exist.

Automaton and *Tyché* are the two forms of chance that Aristotle considered. In the Suite or Exercises, the two are not clearly differentiated and both are subsumed under the principle of the repetition compulsion. "What are you, figure of the dice I roll in your chance encounter (*tyché*) with my fortune?" (Lacan, 1956, p. 28). It is important to 'remember' that in Beyond the Pleasure Principle, Freud (1920) pointed out that repetition in trauma, or the return to the place of trauma is not only a *daemon* of repetition, but also an attempt at catharsis, healing, and repetition with a difference that makes all the difference.

The Lacanian concept of the Real eludes and disconcerts because it is situated in a dimension beyond formal logic/binary language and the senses and yet it is intrinsically 'bound up' with language and the senses.

Lacan links the Real to the concept of *Tyché* in Aristotle. Aristotle (350 BCE/2002) distinguished between causality and chance as an accidental form of causality. In the Physics, Aristotle distinguishes between two modes or types of causality: causality proper (four causes) and two kinds of chance. The two kinds of chance are *automaton* and *tyché*. It is important to distinguish between the two types of causality (causality proper and chance) and the two types of chance because these are often confused. In fact, Lacan also refers to *tyché* as a form of causality instead of as a form of accidental causality.

More recently, after Aristotle, Hume (1748, Of Probability) distinguished between causality and probability. Due to our ignorance or the limitations of our cognitive and perceptual functions we miss many small, numerous, or complex forms of causality. At some point, complexity renders prediction impossible. From this perspective, the most we can know is various degrees of probability that certain events may be causally related to one another. Chance is an everyday word used when speaking about an event taking place while probability is a precise measurement of that chance. In the roll of the dice, each of the six numbers/sides of a dice have a 1/6 chance of manifesting. Probability is a special branch of mathematics that helps people decide the percentage of likelihood of an event taking place.

For Aristotle (Physics) there were two forms of chance or accidental/spontaneous/random causality: *Tyché* and *Automaton*. Of the two only *Tyché* is truly spontaneous or Real. *Automaton* appears random because it disrupts predictable social behaviour derived from social norms but is determined by very precise signifying chains of conscious or unconscious causality. *Automaton* is the disruptive psychical causality associated with the Freudian Unconscious while *Tyché* is the type of chance linked to the Lacanian Real unconscious.

There is what cannot be represented about the drive (*Tyché*) as well as what cannot be measured or predicted due to the complexity of factors and causes at work (*Automaton*). In formal logic certainty is expressed in terms of the probability that preferential states and beliefs will manifest and prevail in the relative frequencies of the facts of existence. Propensities, tendencies, or human habits, "must obey" the usual probability calculus. Objective probability represents the hope that nature functions according to the categories of formal logic. *Automaton* or accidental causality refers to the unconsciously repressed elements that we do not expect (accidental/random) and are not socially desirable and yet remain an intrinsic aspect of the facts of existence. What appears random and irrational may obey and be determined by logical and mathematical principles of a different order.

Tyché for Lacan represents an encounter with the Real and manifests in free association. Encounters are things that one suffers/enjoys in abeyance or pending receiving the necessary attention in the practice of speech or analysis. *Tyché* (as written in Seminar XI) or *Tyché* and automaton are accidental causes. *Tyché* is destiny, and *Automaton* is chance associated with instincts and non-rational beings and their fate. With speaking beings, *Automaton*, according to Lacan, operates within the signifying chains of language and the Unconscious. Accidental causes produce unintended outcomes or consequences. Unintended consequences could be a transformation into the opposite of what was intended or a different outcome than was originally intended. In fact, this definition could also serve as a definition of the Freudian unconscious. Instinct and drive are also organized by logic and numbers of a different order (symmetrical dialectical logic and irrational or imaginary numbers, for example).

The so-called irrational is not so, since irrational numbers, for example, are still real numbers composed of decimals, fractions, infinitesimals that can be logically organized into patterns. Jouissance, plus emotion in general can be irrational. Such is the case in the first two jouissances (of the Other and phallic), but more fundamentally the Third Other jouissance is beyond the logic of the signifier (rather than irrational) and is unfathomable or cannot be measured. Jouissance can be irrational, or pre-rational, as in instinct, impulse, the fusion with the mother, sexual intercourse, and emotional reactivity, although these mental formations may be organized by a different family of numbers called irrational numbers. The fact that this family of numbers are called irrational does not mean that they are not rationally organized. In Chaos theory, the Chaos of complex causality in nature, is not without the 'strange attractors' that organize a pattern or regularity amidst and despite the Chaos.

But jouissance is not only pre-rational or irrational, jouissance is also post-rational or a form of reason beyond reason (Nous) without being teleological or hierarchical. This is *Tyché*. There is an aim and at the same time the proof of the aim is in the activity itself. Human activity is both linear and circular. A line is also a circle if taken far enough. We walk on a line, from point A to point/aim B and we think we advanced or moved forward but unbeknownst to us we also move along the circumference of a moving circular or spherical planet. Eventually we return to the place where we started, at least metaphorically, if not literally.

The Third jouissance is a true enigma, unknowable rather than unknown, *Tyché* and Real more than *Automaton and Symbolic*. As I said earlier, the status or dignity of *das Ding* (the object as a thing, does not mean treating a thing like an object or a concept, but as a form of jouissance), does not amount to hierarchical linearity. As Lacan (1975) says in '*La Troisième*:' "*La Troisième, elle revient, c'est toujours la première*" or "*La troisième… C'est encore la première*" (The Third, it returns, it's always the First, or The Third always returns as the First). Being First here is not a compliment. The First refers to the inconvenient first jouissance of the Other. The beyond reason of the Third jouissance is rendered and confused with the irrationality of the First, despite the fact that the instinctual irrationality of the First may be organized by irrational numbers that are necessary numbers nonetheless, just like instincts and drives are necessary and yet problematic in Culture at the same time (discontent = pathos = passion = jouissance).

For animal instincts, the Third is the First, while for speaking beings the First is the Third. The two are homogenous yet different from each other. For example, the Third returns as the First, in the mystical oceanic feeling that Freud mistakenly considered as exactly equivalent to the ambivalent fusion with the mother. With Lacan we can differentiate the two as well as bring them into relationship with one another. The Third in the case of the Third jouissance is not the same as the Third of the code, the NoF, or the phallic function of castration. The latter is what connects the Third of the code with the Third jouissance. The Third of the symbolic code is what transforms the First jouissance of the Other into phallic jouissance (the Second jouissance). However, the symbolic function/phallus is not only a signifier of phallic jouissance. The property of the symbolic phallus, as a missing phallus, that appears in the place of the lack in the Other S(Ø), is also the access point or portal to the Third jouissance beyond the phallic signifier.

Jouissance "ex-sists" or both exists and does not exist, and neither. Jouissance is larger than these categories and can only be approximated by a negative dialectic or the logic of the not-All: "It's not that," or neither exists nor does not exist. One way to speak positively of the impossibility of jouissance is with a double negative: "Jouissance does not not exist." Jouissance "ex-sists" or both exists and does not exist, and neither. Jouissance is the function of the 'naught' or is on the side of the 'no-thing', and the proof that it exists. The 'thing' refers to the First jouisance of the Other, while the 'no-thing' refers to the Third or Other jouissance. And since it is the naught that we are speaking of, then I can say that the naught 'ex-sists' because what exists of the naught in experience exists but cannot be known or said ('ex-sists') in language. Therefore, the naught both exists and does not exist in the Symbolic order as a category. It 'ex-sists' outside the categories, or it is a word for a no-word.

Even if a computer or artificial intelligence could operate according to negative dialectics (so far it cannot), the computer would still not experience jouissance, whether primitive or original. Inexistence or non-existence for the computer is simply the negative absence of a number but not a form of jouissance that in speaking beings can be evoked by the negative as a presence from which light ushers forth. Jouissance and the signifier are of different orders (Real and Symbolic) but are not incompatible. Jouissance and the signifier are incommensurable in the sense that there is no metalanguage that would resolve/reduce/translate them to a common language or standard, but they are compatible in the sense that they interpenetrate: there are words of jouissance and jouissance within words. But with respect to computers, the logic of the signifying chain works rather well with the chain/string of symbols used by computers, but computers do not experience jouissance.

> Of course, there are things that run and that certainly seem to work like little machines—they are called computers. I am willing to accept the notion that a computer thinks. But that it knows, who would say such a thing? For the foundation of knowledge is that the jouissance of its exercise, is the same as of its acquisition. (Lacan, 1971–1972, p. 97, section on Knowledge and Truth)

Knowledge interacts with so-called objective reality, but it is also capable of evoking a jouissance in the Real. If knowledge (*savoir* rather than connaissance [cognisance]) is a form of experiential knowing and not just information (knowledge without jouissance), or objective knowledge, then human knowing cannot be replicated by a machine. Jouissance is not a feeling but refers more generally to the quality of affects being either pleasant, unpleasant or painful, and neutral. Feelings are emotional interpretants of the words of the Other. Jouissance, however, has no reference to the Other and to the various feelings and suffering that can be evoked in the subject as a result of the words and actions of the Other. Jouissance only wants satisfaction, and after meeting impossibility and infinity, jouissance simply says: "this is enough (*satis*)!". Beyond this limit or barrier, satisfaction or jouissance cannot be realized. This limit or Real of jouissance is what the subject needs to take responsibility for. The subject is responsible for jouissance and its consequences, but not for the influence of the words of the other.

In addition, the intensity or quanta of affect also interacts with whether the affect is felt as pleasant or unpleasant. There are pleasant and unpleasant increases and decreases of tension, and if there is pain and tension, pain and tension can work in the service of joy and creativity, rather than as ends in themselves. Pleasure can also work in the service of pain, or the eventual pain that pleasure will turn into. This is a displaced form of passion since in the case of pain or suffering only dispassion turns pain into something positive like compassion for self or others. In the case of pleasure and joy, dispassion, as a kind of aloof and cold objective detachment, can annul the positive and healthy aspects of jouissance and passion; or dispassion can help rid pleasure and joy of an unhealthy form of attachment, chaotic over-excitement, or addiction to the object.

In the latter case, dispassion turns the passion of attachment into compassion. Compassion is the jouissance of a warm desire devoid of passion in the sense of reactivity. Compassion responds in unison, together with the passions of others, without personal reactivity, preference, or personal freedoms interfering with the freedoms of others. However, compassion is not the sympathy or pity for others that can easily turn into contempt and the opposite of compassion. There are compassionate forms of co-dependence that kill! In addition, there are forms of compassion and empathy that do not help others in the long run. If you give money to a homeless person with an addiction, you help them feel better in the short run (by having money to buy substances) but make the problem worse in the long run. Also, if you are empathic with someone's version of a story or their defences, they feel you are on their side, but does not necessarily help them to eventually work through their defences and distortions. This is why confronting someone's defences, or their versions of events, will remain a necessary component of analytic treatment. Compassion has to be guided by personal experience and knowledge.

Dispassion is the opposite of reactivity and can appear to be the opposite of the false compassion mentioned. Dispassion can appear as aloofness and defensive detachment or can be positively revealed in 'knowing how to' (*savoir faire*) handle or balance relative proportions in particular situations, however unsatisfactory they may be. Within Lacanian psychoanalysis a warm desire without reactivity or object, is known as the desire of the analyst that makes good use of passion but turns it into a compassionate love of unconscious knowing. Unconscious knowing is the place where I find the lack/emptiness of the object, the signifier, and the Other, "as-in-myself."

Suffering also represents the suffering-through the subjection of the subject to the Other and the signifier and does not only represent the suffering associated with the abuse perpetrated by the Other. In this sense suffering represents symbolic castration as the mental equivalent of a necessary kind of growth pain (like exercise). The subject submits to the agency and determination of the signifying structure. Only for humans, obeying the codes and rules of a program can represent a form of suffering. For humans, following the program can be suffering under the designs of others, but for a machine following the program simply represents the 'pain' of exertion and energy expenditure. In this respect, what appears to be an advantage of the machine not to take things "emotionally" or "personally," and therefore be able to display higher degrees of efficiency, can also lead to the downfall of bureaucratically carrying out inhuman orders, or according to program, like in the Nazi killing machine. Suffering in this example, is equivalent to slavery, oppression, torture, and murder. These are all actions that go against a 'Sense' of not causing harm to self or others, protection under the Law, and equality for all.

Automaton is more characteristic of nature and "unreasoning agents" as in the example of animal instincts. Here the connection between unconscious psychical causality, nature, and instinct, cannot fail to be made. *Automaton* as unconscious determination is also linked to chance and its derivation from the Latin *cadere*—to fall, and to fall away from the norm and towards decadence. Games of chance are also associated with decadence and with leaning or decline rather than being upright. It is well known that the study of probability was historically linked to the outcome of games of chance.

For Lacan, the Real is beyond and behind *automaton* and can be linked to accidental events that have an effect on a subject's destiny. This is to be distinguished from fate, that represents a fall as in the example of Oedipus, who ended up killing his father and marrying his mother, despite his otherwise preconscious and socially acceptable intentions.

Lacan distinguishes between lawful regularity in nature and what he calls causality in the form of a gap (of causality). The notion of cause in Lacan turns causal determination on its head and instead refers to something undetermined. *Tyché* as causality in the form of a gap, *a*causality, and the unconditioned/undetermined, is a new and surprising enigmatic knowledge emerging in the Real of here and now experience as a missed encounter. However, there is also a need to differentiate between what could be known under different logical/rational principles, and the existence of un-determination per se, the emptiness of inherent nature, and what may be inconceivable or unknowable by logical principles of any kind whatsoever.

Some authors confuse *Automaton* with causality proper. This is not accidental (pardon the pun) given that *Automaton* is a type of chance that only appears to be arbitrary or contingent. In fact, *Automaton* is the result of structural and unconscious unintended consequences. For example, a person wanted to say one thing and instead said the opposite. Here chance in the sense of change only appears to be something new or spontaneous. *Automaton* is the permutation of pre-determined structural factors. Change or chance here does not escape determinism. This is particularly true of unconscious psychical causality and the repetition of trauma and suffering, whether in pain or pleasure, in desiring the desires of others or repeating their painful mistakes.

Lacan relocates *Automaton* within the network of signifiers in language. It seems the ego has autonomous choice but in fact the subject is determined by the heteronomy of the signifier and the fact that language and the Other speak through the subject. Finally, the heteronomy of the signifier can work for desire/wishing that may conflict with social norms, or the signifier can work for the regulation of desire according to the laws of signification, substitution, and censorship.

Tyché is the more distinctly human type of chance which, on the one hand, represents the possibility of something truly arbitrary, contingent, as well as new, but can also be linked to what Aristotle called luck or virtue in the sphere of ethical actions. Although the results/effects of moral choice appear undetermined until a choice is made, the only thing undetermined is the emptiness or the yet undefined nature of the choice itself. The structure and arc of possible choices, and what the symbolic consequences may be, are pre-determined. However, depending on the choice the results/outcomes may vary and lead to different permutations of the structure. Human nature is undetermined or unfixed until a choice is made and the outcomes of our choices return in the various forms of causality including *Automaton*.

Lacan says that the encounters with the Real are missed encounters or failed encounters. It is the failed encounter with the Real that links the two forms of accidental causality. The Real lies beyond or behind automaton, and un-determination interacts with determination or begins where determination, symbolization, or interpretation ends or fails. The Real unconscious remains unborn or unrealized in language and is realized as a form of jouissance that passes representation and understanding.

A missed encounter fails in the sense that the encounter or the jouissance at stake remains unrepresented as something suffered or enjoyed. When the Real is symbolized, something of the Real is lost in translation. There are the gaps in the signifying chain left behind by the work of repression (the false hole of Seminar XXIII) and then there is the gap that appears in the Symbolic due to the Real (a true hole) being the Being of non-being and non-being refers to what does not have being or existence within the chain of signifiers. Whether this is an ontological or pre-ontological state of affairs is a mute question because the larger Real manifests or opens within the chains of being yet closes and retains the quality of non-being or emptiness with respect to the Symbolic.

Using Godel's theory (outside the PM arithmetical system), I can say that the gap in the symbolic chain is the incomplete or the unproven truth that renders symbolic chains consistent. What is undetermined about the Real causes a gap in the chain that sets the chains of causality into motion, but the concept of the lack belongs to the Symbolic while the lack of a concept belongs to the Real. *Automaton* does not determine the Real (that remains undetermined) but does circumscribe or determine the limits beyond which the Real can be found. Human nature is what remains after automaton or the machine has run its course.

The Symbolic does not cease in its efforts to represent how the Real appears as a gap within the Symbolic and at the same time the Real does not cease from NOT being written because the Real is beyond the signifier. This is how the two forms of accidental causality are interwoven: causality functions as a gap within the Symbolic yet the gap or Real itself beyond/behind the signifier is undetermined. The missed encounter is only on the side of the Symbolic because, according to Lacan, the Real is a 'darkling' or a dark plenum without differentiations.

With regards to the unconscious, the ego fails or makes allegedly unintended mistakes, and the unconscious represents threats to the ego's imaginary self-image. However, with regards to the subject, the Real is always beyond the ego's reach, and beyond moral determinism and conditioning, whether positive or negative. The unconditioned Real does not fit within the structure of symbolic laws or moral determinism and, therefore, like an unpredictable earthquake, the Real can shake the foundations of lawful regularity. The symbolic unconscious and the pleasure principle are organized around a core of defenses/avoidances and wishes and yet the wishes and defenses themselves represent an irreducible core of emptiness or lack of being. Neither the Imaginary nor the Symbolic can render the Real because the Real remains *a*causal or unconditioned.

There are two levels of chance, corresponding to two levels of the Real: The Real as a true and false hole, as *Tyché* and *Automaton*. The ambiguity regarding the nature of the binary signifier precisely refers to the division of the subject. Such division is reflected in the division between the primarily repressed signifier, and the representative substitute which then will become the object of a secondary repression. However, the division of the subject is also revealed in an ambiguity or uncertainty between the primarily repressed signifier at the core of being, and the disappeared subject qua-nothing or non-being (as the essence of the core of being or the non-being within being). The ego and the pre-subject disappears ($) or is barred under the object cause of the mother's desire. However, under the signifier, and specially the Name of the Father coming from the Real, the subject is not absorbed by the object but rather disappears into the Real, after the *objet a* has dissolved and failed to sustain itself (as a semblance of Being) in approaching the Real (Lacan, 1971–1972, p. 95).

The S of the subject can either be the pre-subject (that appears at the top left of the L schema) or the imaginary object the child represents (under primary repression) as an object of the mother's desire. The S then needs to be barred ($) and the S as $ or S_1/S_2 becomes the relation of signification between metaphors, and between subjects and signifiers. In the *matheme* for the fantasy or phantasm, the subject appears as a divided subject in relation to the primary part object of fantasy cause of desire ($◊*a*). But in the ego-narrative of social discourse the subject appears subordinate to the Other: s(A) or s(O). In the upper chain the subject appears as the capital S pure signifier of the subject designating the place of jouissance and the subject of the Real as a hole in the Other S(Ø) since the Other does not have the signifiers to represent what is Real about the subject.

The Real of jouissance can be of the order of the primarily repressed (the jouissance of the Other precipitated by the object), or of what remains of the subject qua-nothing behind a bar that has or acquires a different meaning (the Other or Third jouissance). Rather than a primary and primarily repressed object/thing, the subject now represents the 'no-thing.' For this 'no-thing' that the subject is, the bar now represents not the source of a prohibition, but the impossibility of representing what the subject is in and of the Real. Instead, what appears of the subject is a metaphor that represents the subject and at same time fails to represent or conceals what of the subject is of the Real. It is this failure that is experienced as a missed encounter. The repressed/repressive primary signifier, or first representative of the drive or the representation, refers to the type of primary repression known to Freud, while the absence of a signifier is due to a different form of primary repression instantiated by the fact that the Real cannot be grasped within language and the Symbolic.

The primarily repressed signifier represents a false hole since in the gap left in its wake "lies" a repressed signifier that represents *automaton* or a 'centrifugal first cause mover of the chain of ideational signifiers' responsible for a structural form of change that only appears to represent change or something new. In contrast to this, a true hole is a semblance of a causal hole but in fact represents an absence or emptiness of causality that functions as a centripetal force for the generation of new signifiers out of the unmarked Real within the Symbolic. The subject of the Real, the no-thing or emptiness, the no-mind, precedes the differentiation between language and being and between being and non-being. The subject-qua-no-thing remains unrepresented or lacking in the mark, stain, or gap of repressed representations. The Real is both beyond representation and the very crack, stain, and concept of the lack within symbolic representation.

The Signifying Machine

Returning to the Fort-Da example, and to the theory of the Symbolic as a cybernetic machine, a register is established (within the Mind or with a scientific method), using the resources of language, to record the alternation and undulation of the mother's even presence or even attention with her absence and emptiness. Even receives a + sign and absence receives a – sign. The plus and minus signs associated with the object (the *objet a* and the phallus) are conceived in various ways within Lacanian theory. In addition, presence and absence can also be conceived as polyvalent or at least representing a quadrant with each element of presence and absence potentially having both a + and a – sign. There are positive and negative presences and positive and negative absences that refer to each other within a quadratic pattern of differentiations.

> Though it might be presumed that heads connote presence (and with its positive valence maps to plus) and that tails connotes absence (and with its negative valence maps to minus), no explicit key is provided. The meaning of each sign lies solely in its relation to the other: what the one *is*, the other *is not*. Consequently, no definitive reconstruction of what took place is possible from such a record. Thus, from the start, there is no true or false; there is only the inscription of a pattern. (Brahnam, p. 4)

The apparent randomness of the mother's presence and absence, her comings and goings in and out of the child's immediate subjective world is the juncture where phonemes (Oooo-Aaaa), as the phonological or sound dimension of the letter, capture the first object, and the object world, therefore, in a net of configurations and significations provided by language. The sound of the letter or phoneme points to the Real and to an immediacy of the object or *Das ding*, and an original form of experience that is lost in the system and structure of language or what Lacan calls the 'symbol's conditions'.

A phoneme is converted into a script, character, or hieroglyphic, and the latter can be reconverted back into a sound/phoneme that now functions within a system of signifiers and numbers. The script or hieroglyphic represents a unary trace while the signifier represents a diacritical unary trait or 1, present in all signifiers and numbers. The object now is no longer represented as an icon, or a part-image of the object, but as a sound or an acoustic image that converts the visual image into a signifier. Dream representation reverses this ancient process every night for the brain to get some rest.

However, the immediate link to the object remains as a potential presence within the function of the letter, the sound, and the effectiveness of the structure as a vanishing point instant. A sound in the air, like the insubstantiality of ideas, the impregnations of the Imaginary, and the place where words vanish once they are uttered, are examples of the *nullibiety* or utopia of the signifier. The latter represents both 'machinic' effectiveness and a failed attempt to recover and suture (through a text) the lost object and the gap produced by the loss of the object. I will have more to say about this further on.

The result of a flip of coin depends "on a single parameter: the angle between the normal to the coin and the angular momentum vector… As Persi Diaconis, Susan Holmes, and Richard Montgomery put it, "coin-tossing is 'physics' not 'random'" (Brahnam, p. 4). The angle and the momentum are the determining physical/material factors. In addition, Lacan states that even or odd, winning or losing, heads or tails, are already a symbolic structure or pattern (the articulation of one word with another). Unconscious thought selects even or odd and, once selected, the symbol organizes the result. Finally, the subject that selects or makes the choice becomes an element in the chain that is organized according to symbolic laws. The participation of the subject in the choice, explains why in the graph of desire, the capital S for the subject is a component of the unconscious signifying chain (see the matheme at the top left of the graph). Further on I will differentiate between thinking, non-thinking, and the signifier as components of thought.

In Lacan's paper, the organization of structures and patterns of symbols explains the functioning of the unconscious signifying chain. However, this formulation does not include what Lacan (1960 [2006]) later discovered through the graph of desire. There are several versions of the graph of desire beginning with Seminar V (1957–1958), but I will use the completed graph from the *Ecrits*. There are two signifying chains (Romanowicz & Moncayo, 2015) and the two are organized differently. What he says in his 1955 paper applies to the lower conventional signifying chain, but does it apply to the upper chain? The upper chain is not organized by binary logic the way that a binary computer is ($0 \neq 1$). In a binary chain, 0 does not equal 1. Instead 0 can alternate or be opposed by 1 (Fig. 6.1).

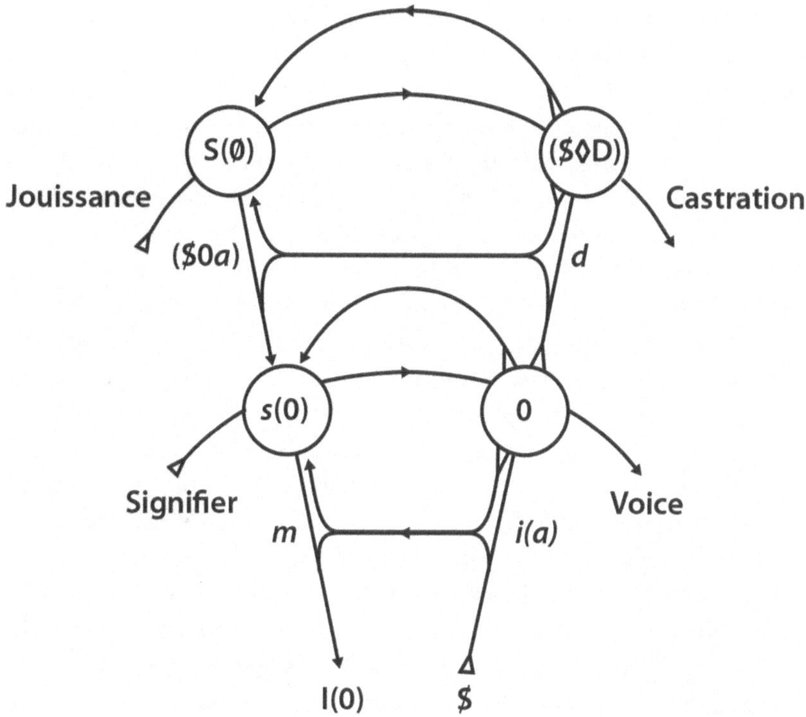

Fig. 6.1 Complete graph of desire. Romanowicz and Moncayo (2015)

In binary logic, a man is a man (1) and cannot be a woman (0), or a woman is a woman (0) and cannot be a man (1). For a computer 1 or 0 are one or the other but not both and neither. In dreams, and in the unconscious signifying chain, the 0 and 1 can be found superimposed and a subject can be a man and/or a woman, or a female dreamer can appear as a man in the dream, and a male dreamer can appear as a woman in the dream. A woman or a man both lack the phallus (1 = 0) and in the upper signifying chain, castration will be differentially experienced as a demand for the phallus, and feminine jouissance in the case of woman, or as a demand for the *objet a* or phallic jouissance in the case of man. But the unconscious signifying chain cannot be entirely or modally transcribed into the narrative line of social discourse.

The ego is involved in the lower social chain of discourse, while the upper signifying chain contains the pure Signifier (S) as a representation of the subject in the place of jouissance. In Lacan's text of 1956 under consideration, he uses the S for the subject that is included in language and in the signifying chain but in both cases what he calls the signifying chain refers to the lower level of the social narrative associated with Preconscious language (unconscious in a descriptive sense).

Four years later (1960 [2006]) he uses the S as the pure signifier of the lack in the Other (S[Ø]). Here not only does he differentiate two signifying chains, but he also differentiates the *Je* from the *moi* (the subject from the ego). The ego goes with the lower chain and the subject with the top chain. The subject now moves further away from the ego and in the direction of a subject in/of the Real. The upper chain transcribed into the lower chain can be handled by a binary system but not the other way around. Conversely, psychoanalysis and the psyche require a different logic that cannot be adequately expressed with the logic of non-contradiction. Perhaps in the future, quantum computers will be able to handle something closer to a human system and capacity.

Signs and symbols, which here mean the same thing for Lacan, are organized into various types of patterns: the symmetry of constancy (+ + + or − − −) labelled 1, and the symmetry of alternation (+ − + or − + −) labeled 3. Asymmetry instead represents the difference between the first and third terms (+ + − or − − +) and is labelled 2. The record of tosses can now be organized in the form of a numeric code. So far this type of formal language or system could be descriptive of the descriptive unconscious or the Ucs./Pcs. system but not of the Unconscious proper, whether repressed (Freudian) or Real (Lacanian). Lacan also widens the structure that is based on symmetry and asymmetry by establishing rules or an ordering of how the two types of symmetry can be combined in such a way that symmetry is mediated by asymmetry.

This would be the equivalent of saying that a woman can be a man and a man can be a woman (symmetry) at the same time that a man is a man and a woman is a woman (asymmetry). It is the repetition or iteration of the codes (1 → 11; 2 → 22; 3 → 33) that ultimately determines the form of the signifying chain in this model. And as if this were not enough, such rules yield additional codes composed of the various relations among symmetry and asymmetry in various combinations. Lacan uses Greek letters to label such new codes in binary terms (0,1) leading to a multiplication of the basic binary level. As Brahnam shows in her paper, there are many more binary patterns in the letter code than in the number code.

"The idea of the binary shifts, splinters, amplifies, and multiplies as we go from the +/− record to the number code to the letter code. What we are witnessing in Lacan's model-system is the emergence of complexity, the emergence of new (unpredictable) behaviours and properties" (Brahnam, a personal conversation, 2/27/17).

Outside Lacanian theory, and twenty years later, Matte-Blanco (1975) attempted to construct what he called a bi-logic to formulate the unconscious in terms of symmetrical/asymmetrical relations. I would not be surprised if Matte-Blanco knew about Lacan but ignored his work in obeisance to the IPA's rejection and ignorance of Lacan's gift to psychoanalysis. The IPA ignores Lacan or reads and plagiarizes him in the hopes that this will go unnoticed given the general active ignorance of his work within the organization. Unfortunately, some Lacanians (the World Congress of Psychoanalysis would be an example) also ignore other forms of psychoanalysis and dismiss attempts to engage other forms of knowledge. Both Freud and Lacan engaged the scientific and psychoanalytic knowledge of their times without worrying too much about conceding validity to alternative points of view. Alternatively, if they did worry about it and ignored the work of others, this weakened rather than strengthened psychoanalysis. Otherwise arguments are not strengthened by open dialogue and instead are upheld by a dogmatic and sectarian self-referential stance.

Memory and the Machine

Brahnam in her paper also brings out the connection that Lacan makes in his text between memory and law. The structure of the language that we use is what allows for memory and reversibility and for what is legal and acceptable within a system. However, in Freud this would be more representative of the secondary process than the primary process at work in the Unconscious. In addition, Lacan forges an equivalence, perhaps justified, between the rules of thought and the judicial and cultural concept of Law. I cannot presume to give an exhaustive account of the psychoanalytic concept of memory but perhaps a few indications will suffice.

> Which is that the remembering *[melioration]* at stake in the unconscious—and I mean the Freudian unconscious—is not related to the register that is assumed to be that of memory, insofar as memory is taken to be a property of a living being (p. 31)…Whereas it is quite obvious that, in doing without this subjection, we can find in the ordered chains of a formal language the entire appearance of remembering, and quite especially of the kind required by Freud's discovery (p. 31)… Thus, right from the primordial symbol's first composition with itself— and I will indicate that I have not proposed this composition as I have arbitrarily—a structure, as transparent as it may still remain to its givens, brings out the essential link between memory and law. (Lacan, 2006, p. 36)

Lacan appears to be distinguishing between what he calls a property or capacity of the living being and the ordered chains of a formal linguistic structure upon which remembering, and the Freudian unconscious are organized. Human capacity, and linguistic and mental structure are all interwoven in phenomena and structure in general. The distinction between capacity and structure parallels the distinction between the physiological aspects of vocalization and speech and its cultural/numerical linguistic components. For Freud memory begins with the experience of satisfaction and frustration where the first memory of the mother's breast is registered. This is also the beginning of fantasy life that later will lay the foundations for organized thinking. Memory proper begins with the secondary process and the capacity for reversibility.

The arch between these two forms of memory (fantasy and organized thinking) is reproduced in the relationship between memory and screen memory. In Seminar XXIII Lacan used the distinction between reminiscence and remembrance to underscore this double aspect of memory. Remembering takes place within a structure and its members or component elements are recombined in memory. Memory is a copula of letters and signifiers, implies a record, and is a mental response to demands of the body and the drive. From the point of view of energetics, memory is an attempt to find a constant name or number or to keep the number constant in the Name. To remember is also an ideal or the ideal of a formal structure.

Memory proper is marked by fantasy, trauma, and repression. Screen memories bear the defensive mark of the secondary process that produces a socially acceptable and personal version of memory. To add to this, Rapaport (1951), in the North American ego psychology school, used the literary device of segmenting the me from me-mory. Memory represents 'meness'. Memory is an aspect of our subjective way of representing the world. I guess this notion goes along well with the notion of ego used by Freud and ego psychology, although not necessarily.

We appropriate the structure of language not so much to personalize language but to include ourselves into the structure that is passed down through the generations of families and nations. However, memory as a capacity of a living being has the fictional capacity to redouble and split the function of memory. Once the ego appropriates memory to establish a sense of identity, memory is divided between the subject as an element in the chain, and the reminiscences of the ego that add an element of wish and convenience to memory. Under reminiscence we remember things conveniently by eliminating the unwanted parts of memory and replacing them with fictions. The 'meness' of memory differs from how memory functions in remembrance and the signifying chain. The difference between these two is crucial for the practice of analysis and for differentiating between truth and fiction, although truth has the structure of fiction, as Lacan says. We can't differentiate between past events and how they are remembered in memory, but we can differentiate between the subject that is included in the structure, and the ego that wishes to reminisce about the structure in particular ways according to various factors.

The appropriation of language represents imaginary-symbolic formations or the imaginary face of the Symbolic as represented by the ego ideal. The ego ideal both reveals and conceals the nature of structure and anti-structure. The ego ideal defends and conceals the gap in the structure and suffers castration under the super ego, but also defends against the Other who can annul the subject. Instead of the capital S being incorporated into the signifying chain, ego memory falsifies the structure by possessing it and attributing it to itself (a false cogito, therefore). This is the key to understanding the question that Freud asked (regarding the unconscious nature of the ego) and that perhaps finally Lacan or Lacanian theory has answered or will answer.

The Symbolic Machine and Intersubjectivity

However, is it enough to say that the discourse of the subject is the discourse of the Other that annuls and runs through the subject or the circuit in which the subject is integrated as a machine? Not only is the subject integrated into the machine, but the machine itself and the discourse of the Other is integrated into the actions of the subject.

> What interests me today is the way in which the subjects, owing to their displacement, relay each other in course of the intersubjective repetition. (Lacan, 1956, p. 10)

> This is what happens in repetition automatism. What Freud teaches us in the text I have been commenting on is that the subject follows the channels of the Symbolic. But what is illustrated here is more gripping still: it is not only the subject, but the subjects, caught in their intersubjectivity, who line up—in other words they are our ostriches, to whom we thus return here, and who, more docile than sheep, model their very being on the moment of the signifying chain that runs through them. (idem, p. 21)

When subjects interact with each other they are enacting, down to the very small details, the machinic structure of the Symbolic together with its imaginary impregnations. The structuring effect of actions may produce what was intended or its unintended outcomes. Either way the Other in this case is the unbarred and complete Other of the early Lacan who determines and constitutes a lacking or incomplete subject in its intersubjective relations. There is an ambiguity between the subject's own unconscious desire, and the structure it reveals, or between subjects' own private unconscious desire, and the plurality of subjects constituted by a public Symbolic order.

Coinciding with the contemporary (some would say postmodern) experience of the fall of personal, social, familial, and political ideals, Lacan signifies this era with the matheme for the lack in the Other: S(Ø). The Other now is barred, castrated, or lacking. However, there is no return to the complete Other of before because now we understand that a complete Other is inconsistent. The Other lacks or is incomplete, which also represents the presence of desire and of the truth that cannot be proven within the system, and yet this is precisely what makes a system consistent. Although now the Other or the order of numbers or signifiers and statements are revealed as having something missing, this something missing or truth of desire that cannot be proven within a system, or the lack of a signifier, constitutes an organizing hole for the entire structure.

Communication in groups typically does not produce its intended effects since, as Lacan says, between people miscommunication or the missed encounter is the norm.

> The first dialogue-between the Prefect of Police and Dupin-is played as if it were between a deaf man and one who hears. That is, it presents the veritable complexity of what is ordinarily simplified, with the most confused of results, in the notion of communication. (idem, p. 12)

In the late Lacan, the Other is incomplete and lacking rather than the lack being solely on the side of the subject that either rejects or idealizes the perceived completeness of the Other. With the lack in the Other, or an incomplete Other, the subject can pretend to be complete and reject the Other or can be adversely affected by the lack in the Other, both of which would be imaginary manoeuvres and results. The subject either refuses to hear or is deaf about the Other's completeness or incompleteness. In addition, the ego is blind with respect to the unconscious determination of the structure or how structure determines the actions and motivations of the subject and the Other.

> The audacious creature is, of course, reduced here to the state of imbecilic blindness which man finds himself in relation to the wall-like letters that dictate his destiny. (idem, p. 30)

Automaton at work in the signifying machine dictates the fate and repetitions of the subject. *Automaton* fails to read the letters written on the wall that determine *automaton's* existence. However, this form of the machine is consistent with the big Other of the early Lacan. There are two features of the Other worthy of consideration at this point. First, now we know that the big Other is incomplete and lacking and does not even exist! So, the big Other that determines the subject has clay feet and may not even exist, yet it performs a function. This lack in the Other also has two characteristics: it provides the empty space to rearticulate the structure and is also the place where the subject in/of the Real can be realized.

The Emptiness of the Other and the Subject

The divided, subordinated subject that is annulled/alienated by the Other ($\$ = S_2 \rightarrow \$$) is both lacking the object that the Other has taken from the subject and at the same time this object is also missing in the Other. The phallus is the signifier of a lack and it is this lack or emptiness that the subject searches for in the Other. In fact, this is where the emptiness of the subject and that of the Other meet. There is no Being inside the Other and so the Other cannot give the subject his or her Being. Being emerges from the divided subject itself at that place where the signifier fails. This state of affairs can also be represented by the formula for the analyst's discourse (Lacan, 1969):

$$\frac{a}{S_2} \rightarrow \frac{\$}{S_1} \qquad \frac{agent}{truth}\ \frac{Other}{production}$$

As an empty agent, a master of none, or a master of suspended authority, the analyst alternates between being an imaginary object and lacking the *objet a* in the Real. The *a* as void places the S_2 of knowledge and the analyst in the place of truth. $ in the place of the Other represents that the alleged complete Other lacks or fails to generate new signifiers (S_1) in the place of truth. In the analyst's discourse, it is the divided subject in the place of the Other that will now have to produce new signifiers that may be consistent with the *savoir* in the analyst and the unconscious *savoir* that emerges in the analysand when the Other of the Unconscious is in the place of truth.

This is how the Other is transformed in history and the history of the subject. First the complete Other annuls the subject, then the Other is appropriated (sometimes without a due appraisal of the materiality and gravity of the Other) by the ego, in its imaginary wholeness, completeness, and inconsistency; and finally, in an anti-structural moment, the ego is released from its defensive function and finds itself as a subject, in the proper sense, in the place of the lack of the Other. The lack in the Other is the place where the structure is empty, or incomplete, as an original form of experience and where new relations become possible thanks to the voidness of self that temporarily (in relative sidereal time) re-integrates the structure.

Voidness of self is another way of speaking of the subject of thought as jouissance and not only as a signifier. Thought as a form of jouissance, rather than a signifier, is a form of non-thinking (*apensee*) in relationship to thinking and the signifier. Again, this is a function missing in a machine. Non-thinking represents the undefinable quality of thought. The transcendental subject of knowledge is a '*sujet sans substance*'. But this is not the same as the annulment of the ego or the subject by the Other of the machine because in the process the machine itself and what is machine-like about a subject is also annulled or found lacking. It is the human subject and not the machine, or the Other not as a machine, that manifests the true undetermined *Tyché* rather than automaton.

To the succession of letters, numbers, and codes Lacan also adds a structure of inhibitions/prohibitions and facilitations (switches—on/off) intrinsic to language that in previous work (Moncayo, 2012) I have argued goes a long way in explaining the problem of the unconscious censor. At different times, or at key moments, there are letters that go missing or that are found missing in the structure and that are required by the repressive function of the structure. Such letters may also have phonological elements that link them to the Real or represent the aspects of letters or writing that bear a link (of jouissance) to a lost object world.

Finally, in her paper Brahnam makes another important point in noticing the function of the missing letters in generating displacements that structurally, and in Lacanian terms, represent a crossing from the

Symbolic to the Imaginary (the interruptive dislocation patterns mentioned in the text). The imaginary face of the Symbolic and of language constitutes this reminiscence and narrative produced by the Imaginary based on the symbolic structure and the missing letters within the Symbolic that precipitate the construction of a fiction in order to close the gap left by the missing signifiers. Such crossing is represented in schema L, as noted by Brahnam, but it is also found in the graph of desire in the lower conventional signifying chain or narrative/story that crosses the vector of desire (see Fig. 6.1).

Conclusion

The lower signifying chain attempts to use the social narrative and statement to close the gap in the subject and the Other. A computer only follows rules and programing but cannot invent anything new without a series of codes from a human subject. Once given code by a human subject, machines can write their own novel codes and create solutions to problems not encoded by the human programmer (Brahnam, a personal conversation, 12/27/17). Human creativity is augmented by the creativity of the human-made machine. But it is the human subject and not the machine, or the Other not as a machine, that manifests the true undetermined *Tyché* rather than automaton. A social narrative generates displacements and a fractioning of numbers. This dislocation pattern within a cybernetic system, generates different symmetrical and asymmetrical patterns that have varying ways of relating to the Lacanian categories of the Symbolic and the Imaginary. Obviously, images are also part of a cybernetic machine or a computer, that like dream-images conceal the language code they are built on.

If the social narrative (or s[A]) does not attempt to close the gap in the signifying chain by using S_2 type of signifiers/signifieds, then out this gap, a new S_1 of the pure capital Signifier [S] (or the subject of the Real) can emerge. Such signifier may trigger a chain response that rearranges the structure of the signifying chain. If the gap or ambiguity at the end of a sentence is left open, then a new S_1 can emerge from the place of the signifier of a lack in the Other [S(Ø)]. The last word or S_2

that closes the meaning of the sentence cannot capture the S_1 of Being, so the said or S_1 remains behind the saying or the statement.

S or S_1, let alone Being, cannot manifest in a cybernetic machine because, when faced with missing signifiers, all a machine can do is produce an imaginary dislocation pattern rather than a form of jouissance beyond the logic of the signifier.

The further problem to be resolved here is how this imaginary displacement produces not only the conscious ego structure and narrative but also the Imaginary as a privileged semiotic modality of the unconscious. Thanks to Brahnam's paper we can now think of the imaginary axis of the L schema as an actual and early unconscious structure that would self-replicate in dreams. In dreams, all characters represent the subject (a′—a or i[a]) through a process of imaginary identification, and yet for Lacan, the subject is the structure of the dream itself, and the navel of the dream is the senseless enigmatic signifier that points to the Real rather than to another signifier or program within the structure. Because the Real operates as a non-trivial hole within each human subject, our machinic structure is still under construction and subject to increasing degrees of effectiveness thanks to a surprising void at the core of the structure. The void as a vanishing point instant within the structure, is not a point in space in the sense of an object, but an empty and non-existent place of substitution and movement for representations wherein structure manifests, as if out of nowhere.

References

Aristotle. (350 B.C.E [2002]). *Physics* (R. P. Hardie & R. K. Gaye, Trans.). Raleigh, NC: Alex Catalogue.

Brahnam, S. B. (2017). Primordia of *Après-Coup*, Fractal Memory, and Hidden Letters: Working the Exercises in Lacan's Seminar on "The Purloined Letter". *S Journal of the Circle for Lacanian Ideology Critique, 10.*

Freud, S. (1920). *Beyond the Pleasure Principle.* SE, 18, 7–64.

Guattari, F. (1979 [2011]). *The Machinic Unconscious* (T. Adkins, Trans.). Los Angeles: Semiotext(e).

Hume, D. (1748 [2001]). Enquiry Concerning Human Understanding. In: *Harvard Classics* (Vol. 37, Part 3). New York: Bartleby.

Lacan, J. (1954–1955). *The Seminar of Jacques Lacan. Book II, The Ego in Freud's Theory and in the Technique of Psychoanalysis.* New York: W.W. Norton.

Lacan, J. (1956 [1975]). El seminario sobre la carta robada. *Escritos 2*. Buenos Aires: Paidos. Originally published in French in 1966.

Lacan, J. (1956 [2006]). *Ecrits*. The First Complete Edition in English (B. Fink, Trans.). Seminar on the Purloined Letter (pp. 6–48). First published in French in 1966. New York: Norton and Norton.

Lacan, J. (1957–1958). *Formations of the Unconscious. The Seminar of Jacques Lacan, Book V*. Cambridge: Polity Press, 2017.

Lacan, J. (1960 [2006]). The Subversion of the Subject and the Dialectic of Desire. In *Ecrits* (B. Fink, Trans.). New York and London: Norton (For an English-speaking readership, in the graphs, I have changed capital A for *Autre* to capital O for Other and lower-case *a* for *autre* to lower case o for other).

Lacan, J. (1969 [2007]). *The Seminar of Jacques Lacan XVII: The Other Side of Psychoanalysis*. New York: Norton.

Lacan, J. (1971–1972 [1998]). *Encore. The Seminar of Jacques Lacan, Book XX. On Feminine Sexuality, the Limits of Love and Knowledge*. New York: Norton.

Lacan, J. (1975). *La Troiseme Jouissance. Lettres de l'ecole freudienne* (no. 16, pp. 178–203). English translation available online at: https://www.researchgate.net/publication/307210365_Lacan's_La_Troisieme_English_Translation. Accessed 22 Dec 2017.

Moncayo, R. (2012). On the Aim and End of Analysis in the Lacanian School. In *The Emptiness of Oedipus*. London: Routledge.

Moncayo, R. (2017). *Lalangue, Sinthome, Jouissance and Nomination. A Reading Companion and Commentary on Lacan's Seminar XXIII on the Sinthome*. London: Karnac.

Romanowicz, M., & Moncayo, R. (2015). Going Beyond Castration in the Graph of Desire. *The Letter (The Irish Journal for Lacanian Psychoanalysis), 58*(Spring), 31–58.

7

Like a Fool, Like a Bungler: Elucidating Lacan's *L'étourdit*

L'étourdit is a late text or *écrit* from 1972 wherein Lacan attempts to formulate his thinking without the appeal to topology, and in a paper rather than an oral seminar format. The result is a very dense and condensed text that many consider unreadable even in French, let alone other languages.

In *L'étourdit* topological figures are found in the structure of language, in deviant sentences that are difficult to ground in each other following a logical sequence. The implicit topology within language supposedly is what makes this text incomprehensible.

Topology is a study of surfaces and of cuts upon surfaces. If you cut the surface of a torus and create a hole in an inner tube, for example, then through this hole the tube could be turned inside out to create a new torus, and a Mobius surface therefore. Language is the structure or texture, and the saying is the cut that changes the structure and topology of a sentence. In this sense, we can use a gap of meaning in the sentence to cut and rewrite the entire sentence so long as the sentence says more than is included in the ordinary narrative meaning of the words. In this example, the Real consists of two voids, one inside the tube and the other at its center. The cut on the surface of the tube gives access to

R. Moncayo, *Knowing, Not-Knowing, and Jouissance*, The Palgrave Lacan Series,
https://doi.org/10.1007/978-3-319-94003-8_7

the void inside and to the space that can then be used to turn a torus inside out.

It is well known that in Seminar IX on Identification, Lacan (1961–1962) uses topology to understand the nature of desire and demand, the relationship between the subject and the Other, and their relationships to lack and to holes inside rims, the result of a cut upon the surface.

A torus is an inner tube (of a tire as it were—or a swim ring, doughnut, bagel) with an internal hole inside the tube and a central hole outside the tube where, for example, the axle rod goes in a car that makes the tube turn and function.

Demand metaphorically represents the turns of the saying around the peripheral object or the turns of the saying around the outside of the tube. I say metaphorically, because it is unclear whether a precise number of turns of the saying could function as some form of triggering or switch mechanism. Desire is the turns around the central hole where the function of the *objet a* is prefigured.

The o-object of desire or the *objet a* cause of desire is to be situated in this hole that Lacan calls the fundamental nothing to distinguish it from the void of demand.

> The void which sustains the demand is not the nothing of the object that it rings as object of desire, it is this that the reference to the torus is designed to illustrate for you. (Lacan, 1961–1962, Session of May 30, p. XXII7)

There are two different types of void: a void within, encircled by matter, and a void as absence of matter and the presence of space (Fig. 7.1).

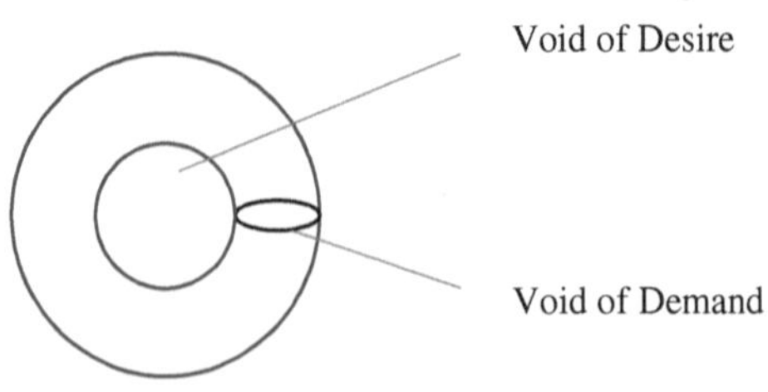

Fig. 7.1 Lacan 1961–1962, session of 7/3/62. The drawing is mine

The configuration/interaction between the two voids and the structure of desire and demand differs for the two types of neurosis. For the obsessional, the accent is placed on how the void within desire articulates the demand of the Other or what the Other wants from the subject, taken as object of the subject's desire. The obsessive subject has taken the object from the Other and fears that the Other will take this object away. Since the Other is empty or void or their desire is enigmatic, the subject implicitly demands from the Other that the Other place demands on the subject, that the subject can accept or reject. The case of the obsessive is the example of an unconscious demand to be demanded. For the hysteric, the accent is on the object that the Other lacks, taken as support for the subject's demand. The hysteric positions itself as being/having the object that the Other wants/lacks. Through various strategies the hysteric demands the Other's desire. Fink (1997) has suggested that the hysteric's fantasy be written as $(a \diamond \emptyset)$. The symbol for the null set here represents the barred Other (*Autre* in French).

The Semblance of Truth

> Now it is…from the place…that I designate as semblance, that a saying takes its sense. (Lacan, 2009 [1972], p. 36)

In a survey of his teaching in 1971–1972, Cormac Gallagher (2009) referred to Lacan's preoccupation with the status of the place where he taught: Places seem to be important to him. He had begun his teaching in 1953 at the psychiatric hospital of Sainte-Anne, he was ejected from there and moved to the *Ecole Normale* in 1964, and finally in 1969 he ended up in the Faculty of Law near the Pantheon.

The status of the place perhaps represented for Lacan his own status in society (psychoanalytic and otherwise). Status in this case would represent a semblance, in the sense of appearance and in the sense of the signifier being what represents a subject for another signifier. The signifier or the Name of a place represents Lacan to the Other (society). One semblance represents Lacan for another signifier or S_2.

Beginning with Seminar XVIII "On a Discourse That Might Not Be a Semblance", Lacan (1971) begins to think of the signifier as a semblance and the letter as Real. One signifier is a semblance for another signifier.

The word re-semblance bears a relationship of similarity to the word/concept of re-presentation. Does a representation have a resemblance to the object it represents? Is a representation a repetition or iteration of at least a part of the presentation of an object? How does the signifier relate to the icon and index, the image and the sign of the object involved in the semiotic process of representation? As explored in Chapter 4, some believe (Peirce and Plato) that an icon or image represents at least a part of the reality object.

For Lacan, the reference to the icon/image is the signifier and the code because the original link to the object has been lost in a primitive past linked to primary repression. Semblance means both what does the image look like, or the re-appearance/iteration of the image of the object, and that the image is stuffed with the signifier, and that the signifier resembles the Code or S_2 more than the object.

When representation is thought of in terms of the Code, then a re-presentation is not an iteration of a presence but rather the incorporation of a presence into a code, where the reference to the object is interpreted in terms of the Code rather than some quality of the object outside the code. In this sense, we can say that the presence outside the code, is neither the image (which is also coded) nor the signifier (which is a representation), but the object as *das Ding*, or a thing-in-itself.

In Seminar XVIII, Lacan worked on two related themes: that the signifier/representation is nothing more than a semblance (1/13/71, I: 9) and at the same time he established a distinction between a letter in the Real and a symbolic signifier (12/5/71, VII: 14). With the latter distinction, Lacan reflects on the possible existence of a discourse based on the letter and its relationship to the littoral (*lituraterre*). The semblant points to the intersection between the Symbolic and the Imaginary, while the letter, as a unary inscription and phonological element of sound, lies between the Symbolic and the Real.

The sense of Lacan's own saying is thus determined by the place from which he speaks. "Now it is…from the place…that I designate as semblance, that a saying takes its sense" (idem).

The said/statement shows an equivocation between the signifier as semblance of another signifier and the signifier/semblance being a signifying object such as a building representative of an institution, or a concern with the social prestige of institutions.

Place here has the topological meaning of both inside and outside that Lacan represents with the topological figure of the Mobius strip. The subject of the enunciation goes into the ego of the statement and vice versa. What Lacan says is intertwined with the prestige of the place, where he says it, and vice versa. What he said becomes entangled with the prestige of where he said it and the triple reference to the university discourse, the analytical discourse, and Lacan's own school.

The location of Sainte-Anne, where he began his teaching has replaced the *Salpetrière*, where Freud met Charcot, as the home of French psychiatry. The occasion for *L'étourdit* were the fiftieth birthday celebrations for *L'hôpital Henri-Rouselle.*

The Question of *L'étourdit* as a Name

Lalangue is associated with the voice and phonation, and the phoneme as an *objet a*, and both say more than the word or the statement. *Lalangue* is the language of jouissance as well as what reveals the buried inexistence of the sexual relationship. This property of *lalangue* is key to understand the use of the Name *L'étourdit.*

L'étourdit is full of Lacan's neologisms. Gallagher states that the greatest difficulty in translation came from two very ordinary French words: "*dire*" and "*dit*". *Dire* means to say. The "saying" and *dit* or what is said, *dire* and *dit*, or "the saying" and "the said". The neologism *dit-mension* invented by Lacan, condenses *dimension* and *dit*: the dimension of what is said.

> The saying comes from where it [the real] determines it [the truth]. (Lacan, 2009 [1972], trans. by Cormac Gallagher, p. 44, 2009)

> Thus it is, that what is said does not go without a saying. But if what is said always poses itself as truth, even though never going beyond a half-said, as I express it, the saying only couples with it by *ex-sisting* there, in other words, by not being of the spoken *dit-mension* of the truth. (idem, p. 38)

The said possesses or is a semblance of truth because truth is only half-said and the side of truth that is not said (but was in the saying) now "ex-sists" or remains outside the truth formulated in the ego statement formulated according to the narrative of the Other and addressed to the Other (s[A]). The saying has been closed and replaced by the *dit-mension* of the statement or the said. The said, being a half-said, both reveals and conceals something of the saying. A dimension is also the dimensions of a house which is *mansion* in English, or *maison* in French, both of which indicate the residence or address of the Other where signifiers reside (s[A]). But *mension* Lacan also associates with *mensonge* or a lie. What is said to the Other, with the Other's signifiers, is a half-truth perhaps more than a lie.

L'étourdit is a play by Moliere translated as the blunderer (who engages in bundled actions) or the bungler. Bungled actions, parapraxis, and the fool are all related terms.

> The court fool has a role: that of being the replacement of the truth. He can be so by expressing himself like a language, just like the unconscious. That he is, himself, unconscious of it is secondary, what is important is that the role should be held. (Lacan, 2009 [1972], p. 42)

In Spanish *L'étourdi* without the "t" at the end means: *Atolondrado* or disorganized, bewildered, and reckless. *L'étourdi* is translated into Spanish as *Atolondradicho*. In Spanish *atolondrar* is to bewilder: the reckless saying that bewilders. When written, *L'étourdit*, with a t at the end of the word (that amuses and bewilders) the title is also a neologism.

In spoken French, it is pronounced the same as the commonly used *l'étourdi*, without the "t", which means someone thoughtless, inattentive, distracted. In this sense *L'étourdit* of the saying or the enunciation of the analysand is matched by the *l'étourdi* of the listening of the analyst that remains thoughtless, inattentive, and distracted to the narratives and statements of the ego. It is not easy to listen to the typical repetitive narratives of analysands without engaging them at that level or taking the position of the subject supposed to know. The analyst is a participant in the analytical relationship, but the analyst's ego is in a place of suspended authority and plays the role of the dummy that does not play or participate in the narrative level of the analysand's ego discourse.

L'étourdit also refers to *l'etourderie* and the quarrel with the irascible little man that Lacan mentions in the text and is a reference to the character Mallet or Malloch in Moliere's play. *Etourderie* refers to the narcissistic investment or rejection of a creative product, the honor or narcissistic injury (associated with work) that can result in narcissistic aggressiveness linked to the fantasized loss of the imaginary phallus and the experience of imaginary castration.

The irascible narcissistic little man bears some resemblance to Reich's (1946) essay "Listen little man" which was addressed to the ordinary ego, subject to prejudice and ideology. In analysis, the little man may represent the analyst who is inattentive to the saying of their patients, where alone truth can be half-heard in fleeting sayings in between the prattle and gaps of the narrative, or in the condensed and displaced fragments of dreams. Inattentiveness can either mean listening but not hearing, or conversely hearing and ignoring the trivial speech or narrative. The latter would place the little man on the side of the analysand, as the source of the trivial narratives listened to in analysis. This is the place where analysands don't know what they are saying or where what is being said may not make sense at one level or any level.

> Freud puts us on the track of the fact that lack-of-sense (*ab-sens*) designates sex: it is by the inflation of this lack-of-sex-sense (*sensabsexe*) that a topology is unfolded where it is the word that decides.

> Starting from the expression: 'it does not go without saying' (*ça ne va pas sans dire*), one sees that this is the case with many things, of even the majority, including the Freudian thing as I situated it as being what is said in truth. Not to go without…is to make a couple which, as they say, "is not all that obvious (*ne va pas tout seul*)".
>
> What is said does not go without a saying. But if what is said always poses itself as truth, even though never going beyond a half-said, as I express it, the saying only couples with it by 'ex-sisting' it, in other words by not being of the dit-mension of the truth. (2009 [1972], p. 38)

Truth "ex-sists" and exceeds the statement. Whatever the statement says, "it's not that". The saying is not the said, and the said is not the half side of truth that is in the Real. The couple is a relation between truth in the Real that 'ex-sists' and the half-said, or between the saying and what is not true, between the said and the half-truth, and between the false and the half true. This relation can also be represented as $S_1 - S_0$ to differentiate it from the $S_1 - S_2$ relation between signifiers/words in the saying or statement. The S_1 of the said is the half-truth for which S_0 is the other half in the Real.

Empirically, the couple also refers to the subject of desire and the Other as a locus of speech as well as to a linguistic relation between $S_1 - S_2$, and to the relationship between the subject and the interpersonal other, or a man and a woman (whether male or female).

Does desire for and of the other/Other go without saying in the ineffability of desire that supports the prattle of trivial speech? People do not speak about their desire and instead focus on the details of ordinary life or the abuses of the Other. On the other hand, desire for the object cause of desire does not go without the saying of *lalangue* as the language of the One or of jouissance. The latter does not rise to the level of a metalanguage of Being because Being is the being of non-being. Whatever we say about Being lands on the side of the words being used rather than on the side of emptiness or non-being. However, *lalangue* does manage to drain something of the Real while symbolic language often does not. But that there is something of the Real in the language of the One does not mean that *lalangue* is a metalanguage.

The Horizon of the Real

According to Gallagher, *L'étourdit* is Lacan's last great *écrit*, a final *tour d'ho_ ri_ zon* (A broad general survey or summary of an argument or event in both senses of the word—argument and event, enunciation and place of the enunciation). It is a survey of all his work to date and a look forward to what is still beyond the horizon. There are still eight more seminars to go, including *Encore* and the seminar on Joyce.

In the current work, Lacan touches on the Real by encountering it as a *dit-mension* of impossibility within discourse. Truth can only be half-said and thus the unsaid half of truth remains both outside discourse and as impossibility within discourse.

Truth can only be half-said and is incarnated in the signifier S_1 where there must be two of them or two S_1: the two sides of truth (said and unsaid or beyond representation) are either represented as $S_1 - S_2$ or $S_1 - S_0$. In the case of $S_1 - S_2$, the unsaid or unformulated side of truth is replaced by S_2, closing therefore the circularity of discourse and turning discourse into ideology, an ego-discourse or the master's discourse. In the $S_1 - S_0$ representation of S_1, the unsaid, empty, or unformulated half-side of truth (S_0), remains unsaid, empty or unformulated, and yet formulated as the unsaid, or the senseless saying.

Lacan explains the two forms of S_1 in terms of femininity. All women are castrated but this is only part of the story. There is a singularity within each (particular) woman that is not all under castration. This S_1 of *singular* femininity within the Real is mistaken for the 'particular' case whereby all castrated women want to be "the particular One woman" who is the phallus and is therefore uncastrated like the master of one which is an imaginary form of the master (the One man).

What do we realize about incomprehension in Lacan's work? It is often due to incomprehension of, for example, the history of philosophy, contemporary mathematics, or literary references, and the use of the resources of language. This is particularly true since Lacan, in his oral teaching, does not present the teachings that influenced him in a systematic, scholarly (citations and references), or didactic way.

For *L'étourdit* Lacan starts with the enunciation:

> That one might be saying (*Qu'on dise*) remains forgotten behind what is said in what is heard.

This enunciation implies three possible significations:

1. The act and voice of speech and the impact that hearing has on the body remains forgotten behind the saying or the enunciation;
2. The subject of the enunciation, that manifests and is heard, remains behind the ego statement;
3. What was intended in thought is supplanted by the actual said and its impact on the Other.

Before continuing further, I need to clarify some terms. In French *énoncé* is statement and *énonciation* corresponds with enunciation. *Énoncé* now is the said, and *énonciation* is the saying. The unconscious subject of the enunciation now is referred to as the unconscious subject of the saying versus the conscious statement or said of the ego.

In the first formulation, the act and voice of speech have manifested as a moment/event in logical time, or as the instance of seeing, without the moment/event of understanding. Understanding itself, non-understanding, and *savoir* or unconscious knowing are affected without the mediation of ego-statements or narrative.

In the second signification, the subject of the saying/enunciation, also influences the Other (as intersubjective other and signifying structure) despite remaining non-manifest behind the enunciation. The sayings of the subject can also be mistaken for the statements available within culture or language (Lacan says that the subject is a collectivity).

Finally, in the third signification, even though the ego of the statement wanted to say something else, the actual sayings of the subject, and their consequences (whether intended or not) still determine the experience of both the subject and the intersubjective other.

Elaborating his first saying Lacan says:

> This statement which appears to be an assertion since it is produced in a universal form, is in fact modal, existential as such: the subjunctive by which its subject is modulated, testifying to this. (2009 [1972], p. 32)

The said can also be thetical or presented dogmatically as a universal or as an axiom. All axioms or first principles are dogmatic except they must be proven in various ways. The subjunctive mode within the statement is what is called an *irrealis* mood that allows the speaker to have their own responses to what he/she said, and in particular to be able to disagree with himself/herself. Such responses are sayings that reveal the subject of the enunciation and the unconscious rather than producing the closure associated with the dogmatic ego of the statement.

Lacan (2009 [1972]) says the phallus/signifier, "hollows out the place from which an effect is had on the speaker" (p. 52).

Words have a hole effect on the subject and in the Other. Let us examine this more closely. Lacan says that a word first carves a hole in the Other before the word can be linked to other signifiers. This must mean that a word links up first with the Real, or with the half-side of truth that remains within the Real, before links can be made within the Symbolic that can be sustained by the Real. The fact that words go through the Real first is consistent with Seminar XXIII where Lacan says that the Real is what links the Symbolic and the Imaginary, that otherwise remain opposed to one another. The effect or stroke is felt or experienced before a meaning can be attributed. The hollowed-out material is Imaginary and Symbolic, in order to make space for the half-side of truth that is in the Real beyond symbolization. Senselessness or the Real, although devoid of content, still has effects on the speaker.

The hole effect is experienced as a loss, tear, or jouissance that opens a space within the signifying structure. This would be the relation between topology and jouissance. Such hole is a non-thought or a hole in established knowledge that functions as a pause for thought and signification. It is in the hole where unconscious signifying decisions are made of what links will be suppressed or inhibited and which ones will be facilitated according to certain codes that determine which information and signification can be handled by the code.

The Real expands the meaning of the signifying structure precisely because the Real is a non-meaning interacting with meaning and out of which new meaning can emerge and evolve. Non-meaning or the Real is always expanding the quintessence of meaning. Such expansion of empty meaning or jouissance differs from the excess or infinitude of meaning found in the Imaginary.

But here a question needs to be asked and a clarification made. Is the statement that words have the effect or produce a hole in the Real, a metaphorical/symbolic or phenomenological/observational hypothesis? There are holes in the signifying net but what about a hole in space itself? Lacan's metaphors/methods point to the mind rather than the nature of matter. There are things beyond the senses and beyond the available methods of science not just out there but also in here (subjectivity). Subjectivity, and the empty essence of the subject of the Real (the subject-qua-nothing) is beyond understanding and beyond what can be observed and known about matter.

Conceptual Mathematics in *L'étourdit*

I will begin this long section by taking a brief detour into the realm of contemporary physics since the study of black holes in physics coincides with the late Lacan's interest in true and false holes and how this theorization expands the understanding of the unconscious in psychoanalysis and of the Real unconscious in Lacanian theory.

Ordinarily a hole is a hole in matter or in the continuity of matter that speaks to the relationship between matter and space, as in the example mentioned earlier of a tube with two types of void in it. Space is a hole within matter and matter is what gives space the appearance of a hole. However, Einstein said that not only matter, but space itself around matter is curved due to the force of gravity. The law of gravity is the key to understanding the concept of structure in general and why the universe has structure and is not just random configurations of matter. Pattern and connections are not random coincidences.

The materiality of the signifier can always be defined according to the materiality of the written word and the voice. Speech is not the same as writing and begins with vocalization. The cavity of the mouth and the larynx is required as a material medium for the transmission of sound waves and the projection of the voice in the articulation and fluency of speech sounds. The orifices of the body, are not only libidinal zones, but also spaces/holes that link subject and environment. On the other hand, speech as sound and the signifier also require a grammar as a system of rules governing the meaning of words and how letters and words are put together. The definition of language is not complete without considering language as a system of concepts and ideas (rules or ruling ideas).

Chains of neurons and neuronal circuits that are required for thinking, do not explain the nature nor the symbolic content of thoughts in a signifying chain. The two (nerve cells and thoughts/signifiers) are related/analogous, yet they are different, and have a logic intrinsic to their own domains. Thought remains something invisible analogous to air that is composed of nitrogen, oxygen, carbon dioxide, etc. These latter three are molecules and elements originally made inside stars. So, what explains the apparent immateriality of the content of thoughts?

Thoughts are composed of signifiers and images regulated by a Code, itself composed of other signifiers, and so on. However, unless words are written, spoken, or thought, the entire signifying universe appears to have temporarily vanished, when in fact it hasn't, and when it reappears, it's not really appearing because it never left.

Are spoken signifiers forms of matter? A case can be made that sound is not matter but a wave that propagates through air as a medium. Is air matter then? We don't see air, but through indirect evidence we can show that air has mass and occupies space, and therefore air is a low-density form of matter. The invisibility of air in physics is analogous (but not identical) to the invisibility of the unconscious in psychoanalysis. In psychoanalysis, the unconscious, as the object of study, cannot be directly observed. Instead the properties and existence of the Unconscious have to be derived from indirect evidence (the formations of the Ucs.).

Sound waves that propagate through air are not matter, only energy waves. Thus, sound is an energy wave that propagates through an invisible medium (air), while the void is not a medium through which light propagates. Light does not need a medium to propagate and this also points to the limits of analogical thinking.

The content of signifiers will not be found in chemical reactions inside nerve cells although the body itself is put together by letters. DNA letter sequences can be considered a Code but not a language.

The body and DNA have semiosis, a system of pair-wise relations, and switches or on-off exchanges of information, but the body does not have the Symbolic quality of the mind that functions according to a Symbolic rather than Semiotic system.

Thought also has non-signifying dimensions emerging from the non-linguistic dimensions of structure. In *L'étourdit*, Lacan is referring to a mathematical or topological notion of structure rather than thinking that the non-linguistic dimension of structure, for example, refers to explaining thought in terms of chemical reactions of neurotransmitters and the like. In addition, such non-signifying dimension is more than non-symbolic Semiosis, otherwise we would be in a circular argument between the mental symbolic and bodily semiosis. Attention on an object of experience triggers a chemical reaction that then is interpreted in symbolic terms, or conversely focusing on a symbol or word triggers a chemical reaction that serves as the semiotic interpretant of the symbol.

For Lacan, (1972–1973) thought in the Real is a form of jouissance that is also found in the gaps between thoughts. Thought is jouissance and jouissance is what grounds thought with the real hands and feet of reality. The reason that science cannot define the nature of thought, and thought being a fundamental capacity and characteristic of human nature, is that thought includes the unsayable Real of jouissance. Silence, for example, can be of various kinds, some of which are coded, and some which are not. What is undefinable and uncoded about human thought is the same as what is undefinable about one of the fundamental forms of human reason according to Aristotle: Nous. Thought includes the unsayable as jouissance.

At the same time, although Lacan at times associates the organism with the Real, an association that would link the Real to semiotic processes in the body, chemical exchanges of information at the level of the cell or DNA are not the same as jouissance. Mathematically, jouissance refers to the function of the holes inside a topological structure, but jouissance in Lacanian theory also refers to human experience, the experience of pleasure and pain, and the workings of *lalangue* within language.

> For the real, whatever upheaval we subject it to, is always and in every case in its place; it carries its place stuck to the sole of its shoe, there being nothing that can exile it from it. (Lacan, 1955, p. 17)

The void or the Real is the Mind writ large in the sense of the Unconscious of the unknown. When the void is surrounded by matter, a void can also be called a hole. The Unconscious is a hole inside the mind that is also the place where the inside joins the outside. The external words of the Other spoken to the subject are first registered in the unconscious hole inside, before words can link self and Other, inside and outside. This hole is not like the hole left by primary repression, whereby the link between the object world and the signifier is broken. A second signifier occupies the place of the signified instead of the object. A signifier is not what represents an object for someone. The object is represented by another signifier that represents the subject more than the object. In a hole of the mind writ large, a link is made between a signifier and another signifier that will interpret the object to the subject, linking the outside to the inside, and the inside to the outside, which in this case is more the Symbolic system than the reality object.

The link between the words of the Other, and the battery of signifiers of the subject, represent the signifying chain in the image of a double torus, one ring with a hole, going through the hole of a second ring, that also goes through the hole of the first ring, thus linking both into the shape of a double torus (Fig. 7.2).

Mind writ large, or big Mind, includes Freud's concepts regarding the structure of the Mind, but also a mind that is open to the environment and located outside the brain or self-centred subjectivity. Here we find the symbolic Other, as the outside of the mind that is also Mind, but also the Real found in the holes of the symbolic net, the gap between signifiers, and/or even the void inside the cosmic web (analogically speaking).

The tendency to repeat, to return towards the same place, returns to the place or the hole where something is missing or lacking and where grief and jouissance are released instead. Automaton or the signifying chain(s) spin around a hole in search for the missing signifiers. The

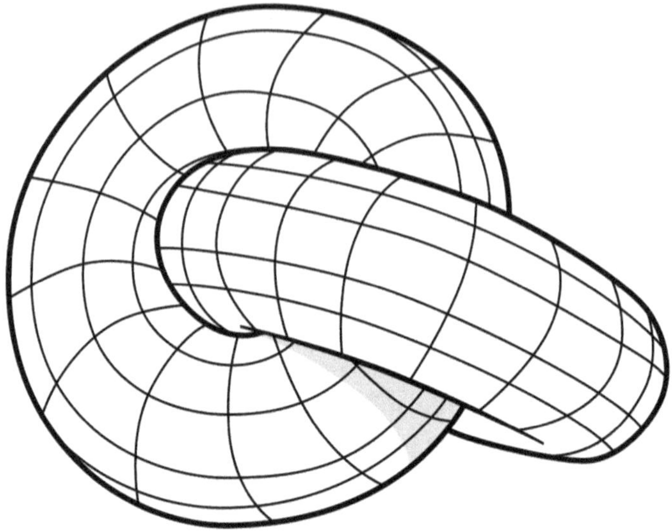

Fig. 7.2 Double torus. The drawing is mine

missing something is linked to symbolic automaton that spins around it, but the hole is the Real as void and *Tyché*.

Recollection and thinking here are associated with the repetition compulsion linked to jouissance, both in terms of repeating or re-issuing enjoyment, and the repetition of suffering. Jouissance, as suffering rather than joy, or sexual enjoyment, is not just an affect like anxiety but rather points to how anxiety is avoided and wanted, unpleasant and pleasant at the same time. Jouissance is like the purring of the cat, that purrs for joy or because they are in pain or injured. Jouissance is the aspect of affect that makes it pleasant, unpleasant, or neither.

In fact, it is the symbolic function and the function of negation that represents the Third of the Code, between the symbolic elements of language, the organismic semiotic processes, and the felt or subjective experience of jouissance. Felt experience of jouissance is more significant than the material semiotic processes found in thermostats or other household appliances (the hum of a refrigerator, for example). Jouissance is outside the Symbolic, belongs to the Real, but is more than the Semiotic that regulates the organism. In the Third Other jouissance, jouissance is revealed as the jouissance of meaning (*jou-is-sense*). The experience of jouissance is meaningfully Real despite being outside the signifier, being senseless, or without conceptual meaning.

Particles of energy, without the mediation of the symbolic function, 'battle' each other after the big explosion or Big Bang, but particles have no pleasant or unpleasant feelings and the battle has no symbolic meaning in and of itself. Matter emerging from energy collide and jostle with anti-matter. Anti-matter destroys matter but matter eventually wins because of a net +1 for matter. Even though matter is destroyed, energy is not, and eventually energy will reappear in the form of a particle. A +1 particle of matter is analogous to the +1 at the origin of numbers.

Something similar happens between the sexes in the register of the Imaginary, or how the structure appears at the biological/hormonal, reproductive, and fantasized levels of sexuality: man uniting/colliding with woman and woman uniting/colliding with man, and the impossibility of a rapport between the sexes because of differences in all three levels. An important reminder at this point is that both man and woman can be either male or female. The relations between the sexes, in this formulation, have something to do with the origins and the pre-history of creation. In contemporary postmodern society, with the widespread failure or instability in the relation between the sexes, and where traditional secular or religious family structures have eroded, we must start from this basic material reality to develop a new approach to the thorny question known as the battle of the sexes. The +1 of matter, does not seem to help the battle of the sexes since the +1 becomes the battle for being or having the fantasized privileged object/signifier of desire.

For Lacan the imaginary phallus/*objet a* is complicit in the inexistence of the sexual relationship despite the fact that the sexes have sex. Between the sexes, or in the sex ratio, and in the Imaginary (the *dit-mension* of the sexual drive) it is always a question of being or not being, or of having or not having, the object of desire. The question never receives a satisfactory answer. Does the question of being or not being, having or not having, at the level of the signifier and the ± imaginary phi, simply represent an example of the materiality of the psyche, of how the psyche contains particles of matter and anti-matter jostling and colliding, fighting over existence, and generating energy in the process?

There always will be a +1 number that keeps the intrigue alive and fuels the system of whole and rational numbers. The +1 keeps matter, creation, and the universe going according to an inexorable numerical logic. Yet at the same time that there is a +1 that remains after all the others have been cancelled by their anti-particles or their negative signs, the process of the negative does not end there. Phi is able to yield its negative image, or better, the same image with the opposite sign. This -1 is needed to limit the excess or inconvenience of the +1.

If the two golden numbers are subtracted (1.681 – 0.681 or Phi – phi) the result is 1. Is this 1, the 1 of the natural numbers? It would appear so since in PM it is used to obtain the golden numbers, and now it reappears as a product of the golden numbers. We already are in a system of diacritical signifiers rather than in a unary numeral system. However, this 1 can also be an imaginary number in addition to a real number. Imaginary numbers, like phi, also have a special relationship to the number 1 and -1 even though strictly speaking the square root of -1 ($\sqrt{-1}$) is the main descriptor for an imaginary number. 1 can be both a real number and an imaginary number. Imaginary numbers have the property of cycling through four different values: i ($\sqrt{-1}$), –i, 1, -1.

The 1 produced by the formula for castration (Romanowicz & Moncayo, 2015), is a different kind of 1. Starting from Seminar IX, Lacan begun differentiating between two 1s. There is the one of the unifying unity (the *Einheit*) and the one of the distinctive unity (*Einzigkeit*).

This new 1, as a product of the formula for symbolic castration, at the level of culture and symbols, stops the jostling or collision for the +1 at the level of the Imaginary. Lacan also differentiated between the S_1 of the master and hysteria, and the S_1 of singular femininity and of the discourse of the analyst (where S_1 is equal to S_0 that represents the suspended authority of the analyst and non-knowing as a presence).

These distinctions are also consistent with a differentiation between a 1 in the Imaginary (we, I, or you are the 1), and a 1 in the Real which is equal to zero. The One (*Y a d'l'Un*) of Seminar XIX is not the same as the oneness of narcissism or the unified body image. In Seminar XXIII he says that the Imaginary and the Real are homogenous and therefore the two can be confused. The way that both are confused is that they both refer to 1, but there are two types of 1.

The One "ex-sists" and is a form of unconscious knowing. In Seminar XIX Lacan also defines the One as a form of non-conceptual emptiness he calls inexistence or non-existence. This is Lacan's Real unconscious that differs from the unconscious of the signifying chain in the repressed unconscious. The latter is Symbolic or represents the border between the Real and the Symbolic. The symbolic Unconscious has to drain something of the Real to produce unconscious knowing and new signifiers beyond those of the signifying chain. What is drained from the Real has a mathematical structure and is a form of jouissance.

I will also use this opportunity and context to clarify some terms used in a previous book (Romanowicz & Moncayo, 2015). A couple of mathematicians contacted me and clarified some mistakes we had made regarding set theory in mathematics. We had confused the difference between belonging and inclusion with respect to the null set and empty set. They also believed that the null set and the empty set are the same thing.

When Lacan uses the symbol for the null set to represent the lack in the Other (S[Ø]), the brackets that contain the symbol cannot be the empty set ({}), because then the empty set would contain something even if it is the concept of nothing. The empty set has a symbol [Ø] but it can't be written inside the brackets of the empty set {}. We could say that the brackets surrounding the symbol [Ø] in Lacan do not represent the empty set, but then the argument would have to be made to that effect.

If the null set is the same as the empty set, and the empty set has no elements, then it's no elements all belong to all sets no matter what set we are dealing with. The empty set is a subset of every set. We could say that the empty set lacks all the numbers contained in other sets (indicated by the bar on the O), or that it represents the dimension of lack within any set. Empty here represents absence of specific numbers and signifiers, or the signifier of a lack, while the null set represents the absence of concepts and signifiers, the lack of a signifier, and the presence of jouissance that together with the absence of concepts, can generate new signifiers.

In mathematics, the empty set and the null set are the same thing and cannot contain themselves. Lacan says with respect to the One that it 'ex-sists' outside symbolic existence or does not exist. The null set is not a concept while the empty set is a concept ({}). The empty set is how the null set appears as a concept while the null set, like jouissance, 'exists' outside the conceptual number/signifier. The null set is undetermined and immediate while the empty set is determined and mediated. The null set is the emptiness that everything is, that is not described by the concept of the empty set that is included in all sets. The same difference can be made between zero and the unmarked, the absence of something and that which has no signs. If we include zero in the empty set, the empty set is no longer empty, because the concept of zero is already the first diacritical number. Thus emptiness (null set), and its mathematical representative (the empty set), is beyond zero and one, although it corresponds to what Lacan in Seminar XIX calls One. The Real is One here but not as a number or concept.

With the golden number or proportion, Phi or 1.681…and phi or 0.681…, as one of the codes that governs/activates the creation or shape of life forms, there will always be another number (+1 in the decimal place) in the series of infinitesimals. To stop this infinite fractioning, and give up the futile counting of 1s, the number must be named. Naming and symbolization subtract 1 from the series: not being the phallus, or not having it, in other words, symbolic castration. However, castration not only negates desire but is also a sign of jouissance. The loss of desire does not take place, because the lack, rather than the phallic object, is the actual cause of desire.

I said earlier that gravity is a key principle for understanding structure in general and not just the structure of matter. Does linguistic structure have gravity? Is gravity what Lacan meant by the material property of the signifier? If we take this idea seriously for a moment, is gravity what links the signifiers to each other? Gravity or structure is what pulls together a mass of concepts and words into a system of signifiers. The concept that gravity builds structure by forging or linking signifiers/ideas, seems to be analogous to the function of the NoF as the key organizer of language and the symbolic/signifying system. The gravity of the situation as a signifier, refers to the law of gravity and to the weight and seriousness of a situation in the eyes of the Law. At the same time, both the NoF in the Symbolic and the law of gravity are necessary laws/metaphors that need to be respected and overcome. Humans stand upright, get up when they fall, and are able to fly. In Lacanian psychoanalysis and the psyche, the Borromean knot needs to be undone and retied by the *Sinthome*, or the NoF emerging from the Real.

The man *moiety* and the woman *moiety* that Lacan refers to in the text involves the *moi* or ego, and the division of the subject into the two of man and woman with a remainder of a small part, or −1, or the imaginary phallus as an *objet a*.

That man is a +1, and woman is a -1, is not a stable formula, because the +1 is favored in the Imaginary over the -1 of symbolic castration that ordinarily is perceived as an imaginary form of castration. This sets up the competitive struggle between the sexes for being a +1 descriptive of their gender. Both sexes reject femininity and want the +1 of imaginary masculinity. Rejecting femininity is the same as rejecting the lack/loss (the result of a division in the subject and between the sexes) that is plugged by the object. From this follows the competition for who will get the long or short end of the stick (phi and –phi). For Lacan, the impossibility and inexistence of the sexual relationship is the 'not to be said' that is buried in the noise of all the things that are said about relationships.

I have been discussing how Lacanian thought raises the question of whether truth in the Real or S_0 can be said through mathematics. Another way of putting it is to ask: "What is the mathematical structure of the statement, of the saying and the said?".

> The mathematical saying, the wall of the impossible (It is easy to make this sensible in the discourse of mathematics) where what is said is constantly renewed by taking its subject from a saying rather than from any reality, provided this saying is summoned from the properly logical sequence that it implies as what is said.
>
> If I had recourse this year to the first, namely, to set theory, it was to refer to it the marvelous efflorescence which by isolating the incomplete from the inconsistent in logic, the indemonstrable from the refutable, and even adding to it the undecidable by not managing to exclude itself from

> demonstrability, puts us face to face with the impossible so that there could be ejected the 'that's not it' which is the wail of an appeal to the real. (2009 [1972], p. 40)

In his seminar "... *ou pire*," (Seminar XIX) contemporary to the text under discussion, Lacan (1971–1972) relates "not that" to Wittgenstein's (1905) proposition that we should not talk about things for which no words apply ("Whereof one cannot speak, about that one must be silent", p. 54). "I ask you to refuse what I am offering you because it's not that". It—is not that. It only looks like It but it is not that. A woman can rarely be the Lacanian version of a Real 'singular' femininity, women commonly revert to being the 'particular' Freudian "The Woman" who "is" the imaginary phallus that both sexes want and lack.

If we cannot say it, then we should not talk about it and pass over it in silence. What one cannot speak "is not that". The only tangible thing about the unsayable, the Real, or the 'not-all' is "it's not that" which refers to the 'singular' rather than the 'particular' object, concept, or ordinary name. The same tangible thing can be said of the *sinthome*: "it's not that." In this respect, the *sinthome* that is impossible to pin down to a single definition, is nonetheless a key element of the structure, and the fourth ring/string that binds the structure together.

Lacan uses a topological metaphor to represent how the unsayable, that remains behind the said, is a fourth that ties a structure of four together.

Does this refer to the unsayable or the socially unrepresentable primary 'energetics' associated with a pressure of jouissance, or the pressure of the drive, articulated by a string of symbols, and/or to the 'binding' quality of quanta or bound quiescent energy that allows for socially acceptable representations to be inscribed or registered and transcribed in consciousness? Put differently, is the alternative between the censoring/censored and the beyond representation, or between the gravity of grammar rules and social rules that hold the order of language and society together, and the alternative new order represented by *lalangue*, the *sinthome*, and the NoF coming from the Real.

Ideas and signifiers have mass and invisibly [to the naked eye] generate an environmental atmosphere within which we live. Lacan says that the symbolic order is a universe in the sense that once you have one signifier, then you have the structure and battery of signifiers. The opposite null hypothesis could also be true: only the relations among signifiers have mass since each signifier by itself, without the structure is empty. It is the weights linking the signifiers in the nets that have mass. In this case, the entire structure could be threatened with non-existence since it is made of empty and isolated elements that only exist in their relations.

In addition, if the Symbolic not only has holes in its net, but the signifier itself is represented by its lack, then whatever is signified that could be absent, creates a hole by the designation. It's in the Real hole of its absence, where a signifier is linked to other signifiers. The gravity of the hole or the absence, or the emptiness of singular signifiers, is another form of the unsayable and gravity that helps bind the structure together.

Lacan's mention of mathematics in the text would require an examination of Gödel's two incompleteness theorems, classical logic, symbolic logic, modal logic, and finally, para-consistency and dialetheism as contemporary forms of logic. What is proven mathematically in physics, Lacan tries to prove by using logic and logical analysis to examine metaphoric, mental/psychical, symbolic, or linguistic structure.

However, it should be clear that in Gödel's theory, logic and arithmetic are inseparable and the same is not true in Lacan's theory. The logical and mathematical structure of a sentence are not the same. It is the logical structure of a sentence that allows for the assignation of number that then can be brought into arithmetical relations with other numbers.

In the quote above, Lacan uses all the terms associated with Gödel's theory without sorting them or flushing them out. What follows is my summary and definition of the key terms involved and used by Lacan. Such summary should help in generating an agreement on the terms, that hopefully would allow the argument to proceed further. For anyone interested in exploring the topic, I recommend a text usually respected by mathematicians: "Gödel's Theorem: An Incomplete Guide to Its Use and Abuse" by Torkel Franzén (2005).

Consistency

Consistency is a system of axioms, whose theorems can be listed by an "effective procedure" (computer software or some form of algorithm). A system is consistent if it can prove arithmetic truths and disprove false arithmetic statements. However, for the system to be consistent there must be at least one arithmetical statement that is true but not provable in the theory. The true but unprovable statement is referred to as the Gödel sentence for the theory. A theory that proves all arithmetical statements is inconsistent. For the same reasons, and according to the second incompleteness theorem, a consistent theory cannot prove its own consistency. "If S is consistent, the consistency of S is unprovable in S." If the consistency of a system could be proven, then the system would be inconsistent.

A consistent theory cannot prove that a statement is both true and false within a system incorporating some basic arithmetic. A formal system S is consistent when it has no statements such that A and not A, being and not being, are both equally true. The logic of no contradiction or that rejects contradiction stands. A or a statement cannot both be true and not true in the same way and in the same respect (Aristotle). For example, in a court investigation or trial, the description of the height of a suspect cannot be said to be both 5.7 and 6 feet two. The problem is that not all truths or human phenomena are organized at the same logical level.

Inconsistent: theories are explosive of formal logic because they prove everything, including their consistency. Inconsistent theories are complete and trivial. This has been an invalidating critique of psychoanalysis leading up to the circulation of a belief, or a climate of opinion that says that psychoanalysis is irrefutable or unfalsifiable. Psychoanalytic theory is not even wrong since it cannot be falsified. If we know that a theory is at least wrong, then this constitutes an advance in science since we can focus the search for true knowledge elsewhere. Propositions cannot be both true and false, in the same respect and at the same time.

However, as I have argued throughout this book, psychoanalysis and the human mind requires different levels of logic for its correct understanding and interpretation, and to function effectively in the clinic.

Incompleteness: consistency requires incompleteness because there is a 1 statement that although true cannot be proven or disproven within PM (*Principia Mathematica*). Such statement can be established as true by intuitively correct reasoning. Statements are true as a function of logical entailment, where one logically follows from the other, and conclusions follow from the premises.

Provability and probability within a theory (letter *T*) is not the same as truth.

Undecidable: a sentence A is *undecidable* as to being true or false in T (theory) if neither A nor not-A is a theorem of T.

A system is *complete* if no sentence in the language of T is *undecidable* in T, otherwise it is incomplete.

However, and this is a big qualification for the use of Gödel in psychoanalysis and the social sciences, the incompleteness theorem does not imply that every consistent formal system is incomplete. In other words, from Gödel's work we cannot say that every theory (outside PM) has to have unprovable statements in order to be consistent. In other words, the unprovable statements in Gödel's theorems are not the same as unprovable statements about religion, art, families, or human sexuality.

What the incompleteness theorem shows is that there is a statement of arithmetic that cannot be decided/proved in T. But it says nothing about nonarithmetical or nonmathematical statements. There must be at least a subset of the sentences of T that can be expressed with statements of arithmetic.

This is the challenge for psychoanalysis and perhaps in the future researchers will be able to 'arithmetize' psychoanalysis using the complex rather than the Cartesian plane. Otherwise in mathematics this problem is known as the Pythagoric snare consisting of an unjustified leap from the mathematical to the nonmathematical.

By proving a statement, we mean testing whether a number has a given property. In principle, proving a statement true or false can be shown to be equivalent to proving that the Gödel number matching the statement does or doesn't have a given property. An example would be Goldbach's conjecture that every even number greater than 2 is the sum of two prime numbers. This is a computable property but it is not known whether it holds at very large numbers.

With the continuum hypothesis Paul Cohen (1966) bypassed the consistency/inconsistency dilemma by postulating two different mathematical systems (M) and worlds. In one world one system proves A, and in another world, another version of the system proves B.

Paraconsistent Logic and Dialetheism

There are some words and sentences for which both A and –A are true. By limiting it to some, you can avoid the charge of trivialism (Priest, 2007).

One candidate for a dialetheia is the liar paradox. Consider the statement: 'This sentence is not true' or the statement "I am lying". There are two options: either the sentence is true, or it is not. Suppose it is true. Then what it says is the case. Hence the sentence is not true. Suppose, on the other hand, it is not true. This is what it says. Hence the sentence is true. In either case, the sentence is both true and not true.

There is certainly a case to be made for the claim that the Liar sentence is both true and false, but this in no way shows that a case can also be made for San Francisco being and not being part of the North American continent.

For dialetheism, the false is the truth of negation. Negation is the operator that (truth-functionally) switches truth and falsity. However, negation and rejection are not the same thing. If I accept A and not A it does not mean that by accepting not A, I am rejecting A.

Finally, we have Heisenberg's uncertainty principle in physics that says that waves follow all paths at the same time. You never know where a wave is because the observation affects the wave in question and turns it into a binary particle that is here or there, when in fact the wave is in several places at the same time because it is the fastest way to deliver energy.

For Lacan mathematics is a discourse, not a language. Being a scientific discourse that is not a language, mathematics is a science without consciousness. But is scientific discourse a discourse without language and mind? If it has mind and the mind is unconscious, then are we talking about an unconscious that would not be linguistic. This would represent another reference to the Lacanian Real unconscious that would be better described by conceptual mathematics rather than language.

Lacan has also said that *lalangue* is the language of the Real unconscious. Since *lalangue* may not be organized by syntax and grammar, and functions more like a string of symbols and sounds without meaning, then *lalangue* could be closer to mathematics than to language. However, *lalangue* is not like computer language because *lalangue* is also a form of jouissance that cannot be reduced to the electrical energy of a machine.

> They circle it as Real, namely from the impossible, which is announced as: there is no sexual relationship, *il n'y a pas de rapport sexuel* (and "*Il y a d'lun*). This presupposes that in terms of relationships (of relationship 'in general') there is only an enunciation, and that the real is only assured in it by being confirmed from the limit which is demonstrated by the logical consequences of the enunciation. (2009 [1972], p. 46)

What cannot be said in language can be written in mathematical formulas but jouissance is more than the electrical energy of a machine circulating according to a mathematical code. In order not to treat human beings as numbers and cobwebs of a machine, jouissance has to be expressed as negation ("It's not that") within the language of the One or jouissance. The Real is a limit of relationship, subjects cannot get into each other's empty singularity, and the logical consequences of the Real unconscious refer to its mathematical structure as articulated in the enunciation "It's not that". But how is the mathematical structure articulated in the enunciation and how does this relate to the limit or absence of a sexual relation?

> Here an immediate limit, from the fact that 'there is nothing' (*n'y a rien*) to make a relationship of a statement.[...]But what is at stake? The relationship of the man and of the woman in as much as they would be suitable from the fact that they inhabit language, to make a statement about this relationship. (2009 [1972], p. 48)

Lacan says that there is nothing suitable that can be stated about a relationship (*n'y a rien*). *Nya rien* means there is no trace of a relationship. The only thing that is suitable is how a couple separately use language to talk about having a relationship, but both narratives don't add up. *Nya*!

Let us give Lacan the benefit of the doubt and assume for a moment, that an enunciation, specially an enunciation addressed to a sexual Other, has a mathematical structure the effects of which can be detected in speech.

The only reference to mathematics that Lacan makes, other than simply invoking the word, is where he refers to Gödel's logic. However, Gödel matched logical sentences with his symbols and then used the latter within arithmetical systems and this is something Lacan did not do.

Now what does Lacan's logic tells us about how the lack of rapport between the sexes or the wall of the impossible is "mathematically" structured within speech. The relationship to the Real of sexual difference or to the Real difference between the narratives about the relationship between the sexes, is something impossible. Whatever you say, "It is not It." Now how does the unsayable Real and Lacan's logic of sexuation appear in the said?

In the graph of sexuation, 'The' woman as the imaginary phallus or the sexual object for a man is barred (on the right or feminine side of the graph) and she functions as an elusive *objet a* and as a lack in the Other (both aspects of the Real that are difficult/impossible to say) (Fig. 7.3). For a woman, a man is divided by the bar of symbolic castration ($) and lacks the object that she embodies/represents for him. This is the case, except that in fantasy a woman may perceive a man as the desirable and uncastrated primal man only to find out later that he is symbolically castrated or lacking.

Clearly Lacan's logic of sexuation explains many things about the differences between the sexes that are observed in the clinic, in life, and in Literature. But is there anything mathematical/arithmetical about this? Nothing in this text gives any clues to help answer this question. The signifier "mathematical" functions as a kind of verifiable/unverifiable property of psychoanalysis, the sexual relation, or the sexual object.

To understand what would Lacan mean here by mathematical rather than simply logic, we would have to go back to his Seminar XIV on *The Logic of Fantasy* (1966–1967) where, despite the title, actual mathematical formulas are considered. For the actual formulas and their

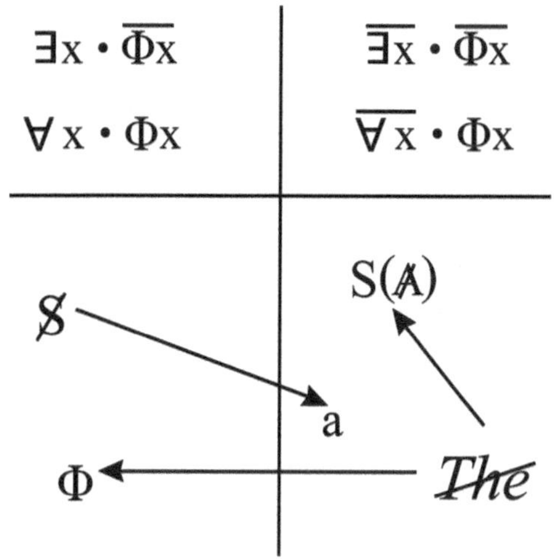

Fig. 7.3 Graph of sexuation. Lacan 1966–1967, Chapter VII. The drawing is mine

computation please refer to Romanowicz and Moncayo (2015) specially the chapter on Phi, phi and *i*.

The truth that cannot be proven in language or numeric systems, Gödel designated with the letter G, and then assigning an arbitrary or random number to the letter, he could use the unprovable within the PM system, but the unprovable must remain unprovable for the system to be consistent. Systems that prove everything are inconsistent.

I am aware that there are a number of scientists and philosophers who misunderstand Lacan's motivations. For example, mathematician Sokal and physicist Jean Bricmont (1997), in their book, *Impostures intellectuelles*, devoted to the misuse of mathematics and science, argue that Lacan's work appears to allegedly abuse some mathematical concepts to describe the phallus.

Lacan used the Golden ratio to work with the sex ratio and the impossible to say about the sexual relation within the PM system or the narratives and statements that people make about relationship. The narratives don't add up and show that irreconcilable differences are based on something more fundamental than the stories being told about the problems in relationships according to the narratives of actors and observers. The ratio of the relation between the sexes is the *objet a* or the object of fantasy that provides the priceless jewel and aesthetic proportion that self-replicates and is self-referential. What functions as an esthetic proportion within biological life forms, or within a biological instinct or pre-determined predisposition; at the psychical level produces an excess (Id = One + 1) that the individual finds impossible to bear in life. Life is joy and also to bear the unbearable (jouissance).

Lacanian theory articulates four different ways to think of the *objet a*/phallus in relationship to the concept of number.

1. the *objet a*/imaginary phallus is represented as 1 and −1 (presence and absence)
2. the imaginary phallus is one of the forms of the *objet a* in terms of the golden number phi = 0.618…
3. phallus is also a "no signified" described as an imaginary number ($\sqrt{-1}$)
4. Capital Phi as a number is assigned to the phallic function of castration.

I said earlier that Gödel matched or converted logical sentences into a string of symbols/numbers and then used the latter within arithmetical systems. The relationships between numbers then could be translated back into logical and semantic relations among language statements. Lacan systematically assigns numbers to psychical objects to facilitate the use of mathematics and logic to describe their relationships.

Lacanian theory uses numbers to strengthen the internal consistency of the theory or the logical relations among the concepts in terms of hypotheses and conclusions. The use of numbers is not meant to provide a proof or a pseudo-scientific status to the theory. If the propositions cannot be established by formal rules of inference, then they may be established by informal mathematical reasoning and its correspondence at the level of conceptual thought.

Since this is psychoanalysis and not the field of logic or mathematics, although other sciences also use them, proof and method are realized at the level of a practice or the Real effectiveness of a practice.

The axioms are not self-evident by themselves but are derived from signifiers and speech produced in analysis. Unconscious fantasies and/or traumas revealed in speech articulate and enact various types of relations between the subject and the object/other in which symptoms are implicated.

Psychoanalytic practice is not only ethical, or practical/professional, but also *realizational* and based on experience. Insight is personal, intimate, and realizational, rather than simply logical or mathematical. Logic and mathematics are being used to strengthen the theory but not to prove the effectiveness of the practice. The effectiveness of the practice is evaluated via supervision or control analysis of the sample of successful and failed cases in the practice according to the analysands' speech and the case conceptualization of the analyst. The rationale for this will be further explored in Chapter 10 on standard, non-standard, and applied psychoanalysis.

Phi/phi are the names for two related numbers, one is larger than the other, and the relationship or ratio between the larger number and the smaller number yields the basic number 1 than can be used to build a symbolic system. This method is used instead of the empirical method of, for example, assigning experimental subjects a quantum of castration/frustration/privation or a particular number for the subject's relationship to the phi or –phi (the object of desire) based on either a questionnaire or a measurement of the sexual organs. It is conceivable that researchers could develop questionnaires to measure such concepts before and after treatment, but this would not help conduct the treatment itself. In addition, the measurement of breasts, penises, and the shape and size of vaginas and their component parts, would yield rather trivial results and subjects, despite the fact that with the improvements of plastic surgery, many contemporary subjects want to increase or decrease the size of secondary sexual characteristics in the hope/fantasy of becoming better objects of desire.

Lacan converts the Phallic Function of Castration into Phi that is both a Name and an assigned number (1.618). Then he converts the *objet a*/imaginary phallus into phi that is both a Name and a number (0.618). These particular numbers constitute the golden ratio that has several properties that are useful in analyzing the logical relationship between the symbolic function and the *objet a* cause of desire, or the object of desire in general. The logical relations between the two forms of the golden number stand on their own and do not rely on what the symbols may represent for psychoanalysis.

(1) **The Phallic Function (symbolized by Φ or Phi)**

A. If Phi or Phi, then Phi (Φ v $\Phi \supset \Phi$)

(2) **The *objet a*/imaginary phallus is the object of the subject's desire (symbolized by φ and phi)**

B. If Phi, then either Phi or phi (Φ v φ)

(3) **The Phallic Function negates the *objet a*/imaginary phallus**

C. Phi – phi = 1

If Φ, then φ. $\Phi \supset \varphi$, satisfies the rule of substitution and detachment. Phi and phi can be derived from each other.

Rules of Inference

A. If 1 is 1, then when 1 is inserted into a quadratic equation as a number for the variables a, b, and c, the result yields Phi/phi. {1, −1, −1}, {−1, 1, 1}, {−1, −1, 1}, {1, 1, −1} calculate Phi and phi. {1, 1, 1}, {−1, −1, −1}, {−1, 1, −1}, {1, −1, 1} do not.
B. The subtraction of phi from Phi yields 1. This is the formula for symbolic castration.
C. If three −1 are used in the quadratic equation, the result is the imaginary number. An imaginary number is a number that does not exist but if paired with a real existing number, then as a complex number, it can be used within PM.
D. Via the quadratic equation Number 1 has a relation to i. 1 can convert into Phi/phi or i.

The negation of the *objet a*/imaginary phallus can be quantified in the form of subtraction

$$\Phi - \varphi = 1$$

The result for the formula for castration is 1. The formula for castration has the subtraction sign for its sentential connective and Phi for its sign.

Numeric value of $\Phi = 1.618$

Numeric value of $\varphi = 0.618$

The structural properties of the Golden number showed in the table below are common to the axioms. The different formulas derived from the relations between Phi and phi inherit the property of the golden number. If a number other than 1 is inserted into the quadratic equation the property of the golden number is lost.

The *objet a*/phallus and its lack (and the presence of the Real) can be assigned basic numbers to build a symbolic system: 1 and -1. In this example, the numbers are not randomly assigned. 1 and -1 represent the presence and absence of a basic part or unit that is considered privileged and important or significant for jouissance and for a narcissistic sense of 'being number 1' or 'having what it takes' in a metaphoric sense.

1 and -1 are the numbers that need to be inputted into a quadratic equation with three variables (1s and -1s in symmetrical or asymmetrical series of three 1s with different signs [+ and -]) to obtain the golden number, ratio, or proportion (form). Those combinations that are dissymmetric produce Phi/phi. Those that are symmetric produce an imaginary number.

The quadratic equation yields two numbers: Phi (1.618), and phi (0.618).

For Lacan the small phi represents the *objet a* and the imaginary phallus as a number. Lacan is well aware of the arithmetical and geometrical properties of the golden number but what is not so clear is whether he uses it as a measurable number or as a concept/metaphor. In Seminar XIV he writes, "minus phi in which there is designated castration, in so far as it designates the fundamental value (Lesson of 16th of November 1966, p. I 77). The notion of value, in this case, seems to indicate the numerical value of Phi in this case. Castration or the symbolic function is instantiated in each case represented by a subject in Culture, and not only patriarchal culture.

Clearly human genitals could be measured, the way that the aesthetic proportion of the face or the entire body can and has been measured, but the results would be rather trivial and obscene for our purposes. On the other hand, Lacan is using the golden number as a metaphor to describe something "immeasurable" within psychical systems. The immeasurable remains so but is now conceptualized.

Lacan says that the *objet a* and the signifier give us the 'ratio' of desire. But can this statement be proven, or is this statement true but not provable in PM? Clearly, the golden number is a proper measurable ratio. In Lacan, the ratio refers to the object of desire, or *objet a* cause of desire. It is the ratio between Phi, or the symbolic function, and phi, or the objet a/imaginary phallus. The ratio between the symbolic cultural-metaphoric function and the *objet a*, as the structural object cause of human desire, is how the golden ratio is at work in Cultural/Symbolic forms.

It is said in science nowadays, that the golden numbers and ratio are found within the very forms and shapes of nature. Can the golden numbers also be found in the mental formations of the sexual drive within human fantasies or imagination?

The golden ratio in mathematics is defined as a division of a line segment into a unique ratio that yields an aesthetic proportion. The first figure is a geometric representation of the proportion, while the second is its formula.

$$\frac{a+b}{a} = \frac{a}{b}$$

The aesthetic proportion can be expressed as the formula above and also as the equation below containing two 1s and x as indeterminate variable:

$1 + 1/x = x$ where $x = a/b$ (the definition of the golden ratio above)

The equation for the indeterminate x can be solved by a quadratic formula.

$$\text{When } ax^2 + bx + c = 0, \text{ then } x = \frac{-b \pm \sqrt{b^2 - 4ac}}{2a}$$

To calculate Phi/phi a combination of 1 and -1 must be used for the values a, b, and c. Once the values 1.618 (Phi Φ) and 0.618 (phi φ) are obtained using 1 and -1 for the x variable in the quadratic equation, then the numbers and their differences can be shown to have unique properties (Table 7.1).

As we see, the number 1 keeps appearing in the relationship and differences between Phi and phi. Whether the numbers are multiplied or subtracted the result is the same 1. If 1 is added to phi the result is Phi. If Phi is subtracted from phi, the result is -1, etc. Despite there being a difference between phi and 1, phi as a golden number has a relationship to 1 in the ratio between the numbers.

The number 1, obviously has an analogical/anatomical reference or correspondence to the form or shape of the male genital, the same way that the female genital could be said to have the form of 0. Number 1 also looks like an obelisk, the proverbial phallic symbol such as the Washington monument, the tallest stone structure and obelisk in the world, that commemorates the founding father of the nation. Washington was the first president of the U.S. and served two terms but did not want to serve beyond that and this helped establish a democratic state.

Table 7.1 Properties of Phi and phi

Phi × phi = 1	Phi − phi = 1
Phi = 1.6180339...	phi = 0.6180339...
Phi = 1 + phi	phi = Phi − 1
Phi = 1/phi	phi = 1/Phi
Phi^2 = Phi + 1	$-phi^2$ = 1 − phi

However, Lacan's argument is not by analogy/anatomy or by using the body as a reference. Is there any meaning in the typographical relationship between 1 and 0 represented in Φ. By analogy, or as an icon, and in the Imaginary, the sign seems to invoke a copula of signifiers and organs. Well, in fact, sexual copulation cannot take place without the symbolic phallus or the phallic function as a signifier of jouissance. The incest prohibition bars the imaginary phallus between the children and the parents. The symbolic phallus is a bar because it is a missing phallus, or a 'not having', or a suffering that facilitates having sexual enjoyment with a substitute to the forbidden parent.

Finally, Lacan says that the symbolic phallus (Φ) appears in the place of the null set Ø. Both symbols represent something missing: in the case of the symbolic phallus/phallic function what is missing is the imaginary phallus, while with the null set what is missing is representation itself. It is the relationship between the phallic function and the null set that grants the phallic function of symbolic castration the capacity to be both a signifier of jouissance and a portal of access to the Real and to variations of jouissance. Because the symbolic phallus is grounded by the null set and not the other way around, Lacan's system is not phallocentric or logocentric as some critics have argued. The null set, the Real, and jouissance, are beyond the phallus. However, if we say lack in the Other (S[Ø]), this lack is both the lack of a signifier, or a beyond phallic representation, and at the same time it also means the signifier of a lack. The signifier of a lack emerges or manifests within the lack of a signifier as the lack in the Other. Thus, I can say if Ø then Φ (Ø ⊃ Φ), although the lack of a signifier is not entirely defined by the signifier of a lack.

The symbolic phallus can also be used as a representation of the female genitals because it is not an imaginary phallus or a penis, and it represents something missing, and femininity represents the empirical reference to symbolic castration as the absence of the penis. What a woman has of the imaginary phallus is its absence, but it's absence is also the symbolic phallus. Thus in my work I use the square root of -1 or the imaginary number (i) as the representation of femininity rather than the missing symbolic phallus. To get to 0, 1 must first be counted and then subtracted ($1 - 1 = 0$). But the subtraction in the formula for symbolic castration using Phi yields 1 not 0. 0 in this case is a real number, that in psychoanalysis and in reference to sexual difference, represents an imaginary form of absence or lack that would leave women in the Imaginary of a real deficit of a penis—an imaginary deficit, therefore. Instead using Phi for the formula for symbolic castration yields a 1 that can be used as a real number and an imaginary number. The signified for Phi in the case of femininity is *i*, a number that does not exist yet can be used with real numbers. The inexistence of *i* is a generative and functional symbolic lack/emptiness rather a deficit.

The unary trait does not have a -/ representation because unary negation does not have an operand: the unmarked is unmarked. The unary trait marks and negates the unmarked. Once binary negation is acquired, the trait itself can be negated (rather than the unmarked) and now we have the emergence of the number 1 and the zero concept. Both 1 and 0 are evolutions/transformations of the unary trace.

In men and women, and phylogenetically speaking, the mark or trace represented the unmarked that stands for the absence of pregnancy/life (0) and the presence of a killed animal (1). The trait is a value that represents both presence and absence at once. 0 is the absence, subtraction, negation of 1, the unmarked is marked in this case as 0 rather than /. But in the unary numeral system / represents the unmarked rather than a present or absence object. 0 is not the unmarked because it refers to the specific absence of an object rather than to the null set or empty set both of which differ from zero and do not empirically exist. The imaginary number is a way to put inexistence to work in a Symbolic system.

Conversely, although the father and men need to possess the phallic attribute not only as castration but also as the psychical imaginary phallus that will permit the biological penis to function according to psychical desire, what allows for the proper function of the phi as a positive sign is the phallic function of symbolic castration. Men have to lose it in order to use it ($p \rightarrow q$), which is the reverse of saying either use it or lose it ($p \vee q$).

Since the penis is not the imaginary phallus, the absence of the imaginary phallus under Phi can lead to a different representation of masculinity in the Symbolic, and to a different representation of femininity in the Real. In a woman, the symbolic phallus, as something missing, leads to the possibility of enjoying phallic jouissance with a man, to a form of femininity grounded in the Real, and to the possibility of functioning as a meaningful non-existent signifier (e.g. the square root of minus 1), and not simply as a token in a system of economic and sexual exchange. The signifier, and the phallic function, represents a form of knowledge embedded in language that gives the subject, and a woman, a safe passage into a system of symbolic exchange, instead of being treated as a token or commodity of sexual or economic exchange.

Lacan uses the symbol for Phi (Φ) to represent/conceptualize the symbolic function and the symbolic phallus as a missing phallus. The *objet a*/imaginary phallus is represented as phi (φ and $-\varphi$). The only way to obtain 1 to represent the object of desire, once the symbolic phallus and the imaginary phallus have been assigned a (golden) number value, is when Phi and phi are subtracted from each other. When the object of desire is subtracted from the symbolic function/phallus the result is 1, not -1 (which is counterintuitive, because by analogy one would think of losing the imaginary phallus as -1).

Conversely, when the symbolic phallus or the phallic function of symbolic castration is subtracted from the imaginary phallus the result is -1. Cancelling the symbolic phallic function produces a -1, and cancelling the imaginary phallus produces 1.

Symbolic castration of the object of desire yields the number 1 as a symbolic unit for a symbolic order of number. Subtracting the symbolic function has a different effect because the function is itself a negative, and this is what makes it Symbolic. The symbolic function appears as a double negative, first because for Lacan the symbolic phallus is already missing so it can't be negated. Second, because the function also negates the imaginary phallus or *objet a* in the sense that both have been structurally lost (-1) throughout the course of normal development. Double forms of negation are accepted in math and other languages but not in the English language. In other languages, a double negative is known as a negative concord or empathic negation.

The golden number associated with the Law or the symbolic function of Culture, or Phi (1.618…), is the larger number that regulates its reciprocal or the smaller unit of phi (0.618). This is demonstrated by the fact that even when the larger number is subtracted from the smaller number (phi – Phi), the function is not lost because it was already missing by its very definition ($0.618 - 1.618 = -1$). The fact of being missing did not prevent it from functioning and structurally generating lack.

Thus, when the symbolic function itself is missing is no different than when it is present. When it is absent, it is present, and when it is present, it manifests as absence in the sense of lack or emptiness. This brings us to the question that the function itself is a form of jouissance according to Lacan. It both stops and generates jouissance, the latter being the positive side of what negation is an as operator.

Human culture is made with similar elements to how nature builds matter, but some elements of matter are controlled differently in Culture via the resources of language. This different way of relating to nature from within human Culture can be represented by the subtractive relation between Capital Phi and small phi or −phi (1.618 − 0.618 = 1).

Matter requires structure and structure requires finite elements that could combine infinitely if necessary. Matter and language share the need for finite elements, and this constitutes a relationship of the infinite with itself. When the infinite goes into the finite, then the infinite is everywhere always.

1 and -1 are such finite or basic elements that contain the infinite and can be used to produce the golden proportion in nature and culture. The basic numbers are used to yield a product (the golden number and ratio), itself used to build structure and pattern in nature and Culture. The missing phallus represents the number or result produced by the system to build the forms of Culture. Culture as a structure also requires a missing number or a sense that the golden number or ideal is never reached (S[Φ]). Too much of this or too little of that, represents the irrational element within nature that is brought to a stop by its own subtraction (Phi − phi).

The golden ratio is at play in the forms and activities of nature, but in culture the number must be used differently to produce Culture. This different use is its subtraction or cancellation that generates a new number (1 − 1 = 0 or Phi − phi = 1). Among other things, what the symbolic phallus as an absence generates is femininity but as its own dimension or on a different plane rather than simply being a negative number in the previous phallic dimension (*i* rather than -1). A woman is not a man (1 − 1 = 0; and Phi − phi = 1). Zero can be interpreted as an imaginary lack or deficit, and 1, as the product of the formula, is both a real number and an imaginary number. The 1 here is not the imaginary phallus but the square root of –1 and the One that points to 'ex-sistence' outside the Symbolic order and in the Real of femininity.

Imaginary numbers or the complex plane must be used to work with the inexistence of femininity and of structure that make structure and femininity possible. This inexistence of structure and/or the decay and impermanence of the sexual relation is the realization that needs to be used, to know how to live within the sexual relation and make it work. Once difference and the loss of the ideal object are accepted, then new words and worlds may become possible.

The Lying Normalizing Narrative, and the False That Designates Truth Just as Well

This perspective differs from a lying normalizing talk about the stability of relationships required for reproduction and family life with children. This is an aspect of social functioning within society that society and its institutions require. These are the stories that are normally told about family life that include crises and the family dramas that we are all 'familiar' with either from real life, literature, or media.

Dramas represent the showing or unveiling that normative narratives about relationships do not hold water and that fault lines reveal a more profound or larger structure that needs to be considered to understand the structure of speech.

> The trouble is that the psychologist, since he can only support his sector by theology, wants the psychical to be normal, and as a result he elaborates what would suppress the psyche (its enunciation and its mathematical structure). (Lacan, 2009 [1972], p. 48, bracketing is mine)

Psychologists suppress/normalize the subject but the same could be said of psychiatrists. Lacan criticized psychology as a profession, and psychologizing within psychoanalysis, something that otherwise might be expected from a psychiatrist. He rarely critiques psychiatry notwithstanding the fact that biological psychiatrists may be even more anti-psychoanalysis than psychologists. Psychoanalysts sometimes behave like some psychiatrists when they use diagnostic labels to invalidate and pathologize each other. Other than reveal an apparent dislike for theology, not present elsewhere in his work, there is nothing in Lacan's intent that could not have been equally covered by the psychiatric definition of normality (although the normal population thinks most psychiatrists are abnormal) or by a humanistic definition of well-being. The so-called norm, as exemplified in the leader, is always at risk of revealing its underside in the figure of the leader of the primal horde.

> the Oedipus complex is reduplicated by the comedy of the *orang*(e)-Father (*Père-o-rang*) or the speechifying Outang.

The court fool has a role: that of being the replacement of the truth.

> In classical logic, when one thinks about it, the false can only be perceived as being the inverse of the truth, and it designates it just as well. (idem, p. 58)

These statements seem to explain well the phenomena of Donald Trump in the United States of North America. For starters, Trump sued comedian and political commentator Bill Maher for joking that Trump's father was an orangutan considering the color of his hair and his pompadour hairstyle. Steve Bannon, a Trump advisor, also called him 'a big hairy monkey' and a patriarch.

Second, considering the Democrats' inability to provide jobs for workers (partly motivated by pressure from Republicans not to increase the deficit—a value the latter have now given up for the sake of increasing financial growth) facing the demise of an industry no longer useful to society, Trump appealed to the base tendencies and racism of white working-class workers to get a Republican elected that will support the economic interests of corporations and the wealthy. The true concerns of those disadvantaged by societal changes, and Trump's foolish and narcissistic theatrics are used to replace the truth of the economic and military interests of white and wealthy Republicans. "The false can only be perceived as being the inverse of the truth, and it designates it just as well".

Finally, the impossibility of politics as a profession (as Freud would have it), and the Machiavellian manipulations that such impossibility inspires, are misunderstood and mistaken for simple solutions that the uneducated could champion by taking advantage of a mood of discontent available in society. I guess this would be a simple definition of demagoguery.

According to Lacan's formulas of sexuation, the proposition that says that there is a one violent primitive man (the orange father) not subject to castration, limitation, and impossibility, is a structural fantasy and not something that can be used to construct anything that would approximate the Real or even reality.

Because of the federal structure of the U.S., the rest of the country could not benefit from the prior experience of California who had already elected an entertainer (the Terminator) with no prior political experience to solve problems he could not solve in the end. It took an old, experienced, and fundamentally decent politician to return to power and solve the fiscal crisis of California. The false must first replace truth, for truth to be eventually realized.

Finally, these political comments are geared towards illustrating Lacan's ideas and are not meant to provide a substantial political analysis that lies beyond the purview of this work. The state of events is much more complex than these preliminary statements can attest. If not only because Lacan's ideas can also be used to critique the neo-liberal humanistic mentality that tries to normalize the limitations of society and the human psyche with an identity politics and ego discourse that merely represents the inverse side of the discourse of the master. A word well said, that is consistent or in accord with the saying or the mental/psychical/signifying dimension of the statement, works better than an appeal to strict word censorship that bears the side effect of polarizing its opposite. What is censored returns from repression in the form of explicit bigotry and chauvinism.

References

Cohen, P. (1966). *Set Theory and the Continuum Hypothesis*. New York: Dover Publications.

Fink, B. (1997). *A Lacanian Introduction to Clinical Psychoanalysis*. Cambridge: Harvard University Press.

Franzen, T. (2005). *Gödel's Theorem: An Incomplete Guide to Its Use and Abuse*. Wellesley, MA: A K Peters.
Gallagher, C. (2009). Laytour, *Latetour, L'étourdit. The Letter, 41*, 1–18.
Lacan, J. (2006 [1955]). *Ecrits* (B. Fink, Trans.). Seminar on the Purloined Letter (pp. 6–48). New York: Norton and Norton.
Lacan, J. (1961–1962). *The Seminar of Jacques Lacan IX: On Identification* (C. Gallagher, Trans.). London: Karnac.
Lacan, J. (1966–1967). *The Seminar of Jacques Lacan. Book XIV. The Logic of Phantasy*. Translated by Cormac Gallagher from unedited French manuscripts.
Lacan, J. (1971). *The Seminar of Jacques Lacan XVIII: On a Discourse That Might Not Be a Semblance* (C. Gallagher, Trans.). London: Karnac.
Lacan, J. (1971–1972). *…O Peor*. El Seminario de Jacques Lacan, Libro 19. Buenos Aires: Paidos.
Lacan, J. (2009 [1972]). *L'étourdit. The Letter, 41*, 31–80.
Lacan, J. (2012 [1972]). *El Atolondradicho. Otros Escritos* (pp. 473–522). Buenos Aires: Paidos.
Lacan, J. (1998 [1972–1973]). *The Seminar of Jacques Lacan XX: On Feminine Sexuality or the Limits of Love and Knowledge*. New York: Norton.
Romanowicz, M., & Moncayo, R. (2015). Going Beyond Castration in the Graph of Desire. *The Letter (The Irish Journal for Lacanian Psychoanalysis), 58*(Spring), 31–58.
Priest, G. (2007). Paraconsistency and Dialetheism. In *Handbook of the History of Logic: The Many Valued and Nonmonotonic Turn in Logic* (Vol. 1, pp. 129–204). Amsterdam: Elsevier.
Reich, W. (1946). *Listen Little Man*. New York: Farrar, Straus and Giroux.
Sokal, A., & Bricmont, J. (1997). *Impostures intellectuelles*. Paris: Odile Jacob.
Wittgenstein, L. (2005 [1905]). *Tractatus Logico-Philosophical*. Translated from the German by Alfred Nordmann. Cambridge: Cambridge University Press.

8

The Rise and Fall of Cognition and the Realization of the Larger Mind of Unconscious Knowing (*Savoir*)

The One is the realization or knowing larger than the subject: The Unconscious in so far as it "ex-sists."

Unconscious knowing is the Real as the One-all-alone at the place where one would speak of a relationship.

Frege returns to the conception of the empty concept, to which no object belongs. The empty concept is the concept not of nothingness, which is a concept, but of inexistence or non-existence…The monad as the One is the (mo)nada in Spanish as emptiness.

Lacan (1971a, b), Seminar XIX, …ou pire.

I will start out by circling around two questions regarding the nature of cognition and thinking. Freudian psychoanalysis has come under attack for emphasizing insight (that people conceive as a form of intellectual discrimination/explanation) over emotional catharsis and supposedly, thereby, privileging the mind over the body. Such critique predictably comes from quarters that given the bifurcation and duality between thinking and emotion, body and mind, chose emotion over thought, and body over mind.

R. Moncayo, *Knowing, Not-Knowing, and Jouissance*, The Palgrave Lacan Series,
https://doi.org/10.1007/978-3-319-94003-8_8

However, the critique of the mind, of the head and thinking, does not consider the different levels of language/speech and cognition that are at play in life and analysis. Cognition refers to thinking with language and to discursive statements that are made in psychotherapy and analysis. However, patient's narratives and statements are not the object and purpose of analysis. The unconscious saying is the object of analysis while the said statements and narratives (the object of psychotherapy) are the carbon in which the diamond of the unconscious signifying chain is embedded.

Two questions arise in response to this. Clearly narrative stories and ego statements are forms of cognition but what about speech and the unconscious saying? If the latter are forms of cognition how do they differ from ego statements? Statements and narratives represent $S_1 - S_2$ relations between signifiers while the unconscious saying represents an $S_1 - S_0$ relation. In $S_1 - S_2$ relations meaning comes from the relationship between words, while in the $S_1 - S_0$ relation, meaning or significance, in this case, comes from the infusion or evocation of a form of jouissance. Instead of the subject (S_1) being represented by another signifier (S_2), the subject is a single signifier in the place of jouissance as an unmarked state or original form of experience that could be traumatic or therapeutic. Both type of relations represents the root of cognition, the capacity to differentiate this from that, and the system of language from the Real that lies outside language.

The perception/cognition of reality statements is equally real and unreal. As far as reality and the reality ego are concerned, the Real may appear as something ominous, painful, hazardous/traumatic, and uncanny; or as something beneficial, auspicious, or even sublime.

According to Freud we experience external 'reality' as either realizing or frustrating/negating desire and the subject. In either case a subject is required to experience reality. Mind and consciousness, in turn, are based on two kinds of subjective desire: desire for objects of the senses (including people), and desire for knowledge or the signifiers of conceptualization. Both can be experienced as something that reality and the Other may oppose, or as something that can give access to reality and the Real.

The objects of knowledge and of the senses are steered by the different forms of the *objet a* cause of desire. What the cause of desire, the objects of the senses, and knowledge, have in common according to Lacan is the golden ratio. Natural forms are organized by the golden ratio, the golden ratio itself is an object of knowledge, and for Lacan the object of fantasy is also the phi number. The *objet a* is the first object cause of desire. The subject is first an object cause of the mother's desire and the mother/breast is the first *objet a* of the child. In the a – a′ Imaginary axis of the L schema the child is situated as an object and this serves as a structural example of how subject and object arise together and intermingle. Both the subject's desire and its objects arise together.

Desire in the form of grasping, even the grasping reflex as a vestigial trait, describes the kinetic energy of clinging attachment and desire for the objects of desire. The desire for conceptual objects and words/signifiers is required for the apprehension and structuring of the world and begins with the act of Naming and the establishment of language. The desire for conceptual signifiers/objects refers to cognitions of being and non-being: thinking, not thinking, and non-thinking. This desire for speech and Names differs from the desire caused by the object of desire, if anything because the Naming of the object inscribes the object in a different dimension of experience associated with the Symbolic.

The perception of reality is unreal because how we perceive is not what we perceive.

> I am, of course, aware of the importance of imaginary impregnations (*Prägung*) in the partializations of the symbolic alternative that give the symbolic chain its appearance. (Lacan, 1956, p. 6)

We perceive with our imagination so at least half of perception is an imaginary form of fiction and therefore unreal. Structure or interdependence, whether in the atom, cell, organism, number theory, or the battery of signifiers as the symbolic alternative, is also non-existent in the sense that they are categories of perception and intelligibility subject to imaginary impregnations.

The signifying units themselves, or the signifier has no meaning or is non-existent, or 'ex-sists,' other than being a combination, displacement or condensation of the battery of signifiers. There are signifiers that both exist and do not exist. Conceptual categories are categories of cognition ($S_1 - S_2$) and not necessarily of the reality object. The object before language is lost when named in the pre-history of the subject. When we perceive an object what we see is its mark, signifier, or designation: this is how the object is perceived and apprehended by the symbolic net.

Conceptual symbolic structures are unconscious at least in a descriptive sense, because they are categories of cognition and are not necessarily found within the objects of perception. In perception, the Unconscious appears not to exist, or 'ex-sists' with respect to how the structure appears in visual perception. By the same token the unconscious signifying chain 'ex-sists' or appears not to exist in how meaning appears within the social narrative. The structure is also denied and made unconscious by how it appears in the Imaginary of visual perception.

Are the forms of nature found in the structure of perception also known as the 'eye of the beholder', or in the things themselves? This question may be impossible to answer because language cannot be unlearned. Obviously, if the structure of the senses is intact, sense input is received regardless of perceptual and linguistic structure. In the case of brain damage leading to agnosia the subject cannot recognize the form of objects in the environment. The latter seems to point to the fact that the golden proportion may be part of the structure of perception or may operate both in DNA and molecular structure leading to the forms of nature within the structure of perception.

Perception is something that takes place within the Borromean knot or the different dimensions/strands/cords/lines of experience as well as across Freud's three metapsychological systems described in chapter one. The perceiving subject perceives according to Symbolic mental categories, how things are perceived as objects is the Imaginary, and the thing-in-itself or *das Ding* is the Real that can either be the fantasy or phantasm as 'the thing' that does not exist, or the 'no-thing' that is both an absence and a presence. The three cords support one another in the Borromean knot.

Even if structures are found in the object, structures do not appear the way they function. For example, *objet a* is the cause of desire but the cause only appears in disguise or fantasy or as a co-incidence of desire and the objects of the senses. In the example of romantic love, narcissistic love appears in the form of an infatuation with the other. The subject believes in its objects as if the object was a quality of the other. In fact, there is no rapport between the sexes because the object is never of the other but only of the subject. Once the bubble of unity with the romantic object bursts, and the absence of the sexual relation is realized, what remains is the One-all-alone (*Il y a de l'Un or Yad'lun Tout-seul*). Aloneness or solitude, however, do not impede or preclude a relation with the Other.

Nature relies on the cultural signifiers of desire for reproduction but the very thing that leads us to reproduce (sexual love) is what causes the absence of a sexual relation or the absence of harmony within a relationship. The structure of a relationship does not exist the way it appears, and the structure is itself denied by the way it appears. Structure is what exists by not-being or appearing absent from the phenomenal forms or conditions in which it appears.

The structure may appear as positive or negative, true thinking and false thinking, visual objects and signifiers, presence and absence of relations, facilitations and inhibitions, symmetrical or asymmetrical, functional or dysfunctional events. Depending on the initial conditions, the elements of the structure may combine and result in health or illness, union or separation, and both can be positive or negative, problems or solutions, or an alternation and sequence between the two.

The Symbolic is the access to the Real and to what 'ex-sists' by non-being or inexistence and this is the Real or the Real aspect of the Symbolic as a hole. Symbolic categories are substantial in the metaphoric (symbolic) sense and yet empty and without substance. Interdependent symbolic categories appear as imaginary conditions that vanish into thin air. The going on being, the ongoing being, and the One's own non-being, are all zero, not going anywhere, and always remain in the same place.

Whether fictional, or symbolically effective, unreal events have their effects.

The Real also refers to the absence of cognitions, to non-thinking, and to a thought or S_1 that is a form of jouissance unlinked to other thoughts/signifiers that could generate a semblance or an imaginary apprehension. Forms of jouissance supersede chains of thinking and various forms of logical connectives. But jouissance is something more beneficial than simply the immediate pleasurable apprehension of the world via the senses and their objects.

In fact, jouissance is defined by being more (*encore*) than itself. Excitement leads to surplus jouissance that carries the mark of its own prohibition given that the re-union with the mother is impossible. The jouissance with the m/Other becomes something impossible that ushers forth the manifestation and transformation of the jouissance of the Other into phallic jouissance.

Psychoanalysis has known for a while that thought can become or be something pathological. So much so that intellectualization appears on the official list of basic defense mechanisms compiled by Anna Freud (1936). Thought disturbance is involved in most if not all disorders. The same could be said of affects. In fact, precisely combining these two ideas (thought and mood disturbance), Aaron Beck (1967) developed cognitive behavioral therapy as an off-shoot of psychoanalysis. According to CBT, disturbance of affects such as depression and anxiety are determined by faulty cognitions. Almost like an experimental researcher, the cognitive behavioral therapist is involved in showing the patient that their cognitions are false. This could be another version of reality testing.

But is there such a thing as normal thinking? Consider for example, that several of the most gifted mathematicians (the Queen of the Sciences) at the turn of the twentieth century displayed symptoms of abnormal thinking (Cantor, Boltzman, Gödel). The abnormal becomes the normal and the normal can also be abnormal. The normal becomes abnormal when the norm, or the climate of opinion that represents most people, becomes primarily semblance or the mask of a false self. Now this does not mean that there is a true self behind the mask but only that there is a lack of an imaginary self/ego that functions as what binds or holds the structure together. It is the gap where the ego would be, that functions as what binds or holds the structure together, rather than the ego. With the mask or normative semblance, the conflicts are simply kept hidden and repressed (in traditional character) or revealed and acted out as is happening nowadays in contemporary versions of neurosis.

But to be fair, Freud and particularly Breuer, believed in a basic pair of forms of energy that are still relevant in physics today. Free and bound energy were the psychoanalytic terms they used to nominate potential and kinetic energy in science.

For Freud, these two forms of energy, free and bound or quiescent energy, functioned in two different modalities of thinking: the primary and secondary process. But Freud had a negative view of what freedom and the primary process entailed. In both cases these were chaotic and primitive events. Psychopathology simply relives the primitive conditions the species encountered early on in evolution. For Freud freedom was disorder and only possible within form or in a quiescent state. Freedom represents free energy flows towards discharge in the most direct and immediate way possible. No mediation here means not postponing impulses and discharging them in the present moment as if there was no tomorrow and the consequences did not matter.

This is something that can take place both at the level of thought in mania (flight of ideas) and psychoses (loose associations) and at the level of action in perversion and drug addiction. Energy flows from idea to idea in such a frenetic way that no reflection or memory becomes possible. However, the primary process can also be experienced in the normal phenomenon of the stream of consciousness wherein thoughts, memories, and fantasies, flash through the mind without interruption. Under stress or conflict conditions or in the phenomenon of romantic and sexual love the stream of consciousness becomes specially pronounced. The same can be said of writing in what has been called a 'fevered' stream of thinking.

Reflection in the sense of thought, and reflection in the sense of the reflection of light on a surface (a mirror or solar panel, for example) requires smaller amounts of energy in a quiescent state capable of mobility, displacement, retention, application, and condensation at the same time. Freedom here means applied energy within form that characterizes the emancipatory ideals of civilization. This is what meditation means in the West: applied thought and the contemplation of the first principles or thinking that takes place at the origin of Being.

But applied thought with low levels of kinetic energy requires periodic and frequent absorption of kinetic energy back into potential quiescent energy that can then flow back out again into the movement of thought, and so on and so forth (The outflow-inflow movement of waves and the ocean would be an example of this).

In this regard, it is important to note that breathing as a form of hearing can have a significant impact by slowing down the process of thought and the same can be said of the practice of writing. Breathing and writing are joined under what is known as inspiration and aspiration. Writing functions as a support for thinking because the energy and representational or linguistic element of thought is transformed into letters in a bound and luminous quiescent state reflecting the stability of the clear sheet/state. It is this form of energy that lends writing, thinking, and a text, the quality of being inspired or imposed by a larger force than the ego.

The clear sheet/state represents the awareness that is a non-thought and a state of non-perception given that no objects or concepts stick to the screen. On the other hand, such non-perception allows for new perceptions to arise because the representations/concepts already established in the encrypted layer of the mind do not saturate the clear state of mind. In addition, a non-thought can also become a thought that has the internal consistency and beauty of the forms of nature.

Symbolic thought requires Nomination (as a symbolic/real link) to follow the golden proportion of nature, rather than simply the order of irrational numbers in the forms of nature. For example, the forms of the leaves of a plant that branch out rather than being arranged one on top of another. Branching in plants is regulated by the fractioning of irrational numbers and is designed to maximize the reception of light and water. Irrational golden numbers function differently in thought given that the mere fractioning of thinking can lead to chaotic thinking as a primordial form of thinking seen in the primary process. The golden proportion in symbolic thought requires the intervention of Nomination to accede to a more evolved form of thinking in culture.

The clear state is also a meditative state of mind that represents a fertile ground for the seeds of thought to flower and bloom. Potential base energy is a form of jouissance that represents a preparatory or incubation state for thought and creation. Thus, Lacan could say that thought is a form of jouissance. Jouissance in thought is like water that becomes a wave, and like the wave of energy that transforms into a particle (mass) when held under observation or awareness.

The absence or presence of cognitions can have negative or positive effects. For example, does the absence of cognition signify the absence of (false) cognition or the absence of higher-level thinking? In the latter respect, the subject can say: "What was I thinking" or "I wasn't thinking". I wasn't thinking means I was not thinking quiescent thoughts and instead the primary process ruled thinking. In this case, thinking led to ignorance or to ignoring the entailment and consequence of thoughts that is the hallmark of rational thinking.

Finally, ignorance can also mean the refusal to think and the wish to keep things simple and unreal while ignoring the Real structure of thought according to which things function. As can be ascertained, the cessation of thought in the example of not thinking is not necessarily beneficial. By not thinking, balance, homeostasis, or equilibrium is maintained yet such balance prevents the further evolution of the subject and the structure. A fixed view or opinion, of self and others, becomes stagnant under the condition known as either thinking or not thinking. If left undisturbed, fixed views and prejudicial opinions proliferate under the banner of 'not-thinking' or the rejection of thought.

Thus, the absence of ego-cogitation generates both ignorance and true thinking. Ignorance because of the absence of reflexive thought, and ignorance because stereotyped forms of thinking prevent the emergence of true creative thought. Creative thought requires both non-thinking (as opposed to not thinking) and a quiescent and luminescent form of energy that links thinking to the Real of the jouissance of meaning as defined by Lacan in *La Troisieme*.

That the cessation of cognitions leads to ignorance and is not Real, and the opposite proposition that the continuation of cognition does not only not lead to ignorance but establishes the sense of reality, are both true. Cognition does not necessarily lead to ignorance but neither does it lead to unconscious knowledge or unknown knowing. Unknown knowing is a primary form of thinking that differs both from the primary process and the secondary process when the latter is conceived as a lukewarm and substitutive form of thinking. Unconscious knowing has the intensity of the primary process and yet a sense of freedom that is only possible with bound or quiescent energy. This form of thinking at the gateway of the unconscious and the origin of Being characterizes both meditative/mathematical thinking and the function of free association in psychoanalysis.

In analysis, the cessation of cognition or discursive speech eliminates the semblance of how things appear, to give way to a more fundamental saying emerging from the Unconscious that does not ignore the interdependent conditions at work in the subject and subjectivity. A narrative, or story-line, as a semblance of psychical structure, at once reveals the emptiness of the Real structure that allows the structure to be misrepresented, while the structure is revealed in the interstices of the statement or narrative. If the saying is repressed, then both the knowing of the structure and of the Real may be missed.

Free association links the statement to a saying that makes fresh new connections leading to the transformation of energy, jouissance, and affective states. Free association in analysis does not exactly correspond to how Freud described the free energy of the primary process. I submit that these represent two different forms of freedom.

What leads to the emptiness of the structure is not the stopping of false cognition but rather the recognition that constructions are not/naught (how they appear in the Imaginary). That constructions are not/naught is equivalent to how a slip of the tongue or a parapraxis, as a saying, contradicts the narratives/stories/statements of the ego and yet the saying appears and disappears, allowing the semblance to define reality. The analytical function is the support for the saying that places the semblance in a new light.

Now why does Lacan (1971c) in the later years refer to the signifier as semblance, a formulation that seems to downgrade and place the Symbolic on a par with the Imaginary? The Imaginary is how the structure appears, while the interdependent symbolic structure is unconscious and not/naught because of its emptiness, and this makes it Real. The Symbolic is what gives access to the Real while the Imaginary is how the Symbolic appears as semblance.

Emptiness or interdependence 'ex-sists' within an imaginary construction and within the structure that is not. Therefore, a tentative response can be given to the question whether some cognitions are true, and some are not, depending on whether the subject matter is the non-being of cognitions or the realization of non-being. Cognitions are not, but the realization of non-being is. The world and many of its stories are unreal. Yet in its non-being the world is not unreal because liberation is realized.

The world appears as real because its non-being also it is not. Out of the place of non-being and lack, fantasies are generated and constructed because, after all, truth has the structure of fiction, as Lacan said.

Cessation of false cognition means not solely the elimination of faulty constructions, but the more general realization that emptiness "ex-sists" in all relative constructions. The unreality of the object, its non-being, itself is not/naught/a knot. Emptiness 'ex-sists' in the construction.

The reality of the subject or the object is its constructed own-being (Imaginary) out of the lack of inherent nature (Real). The unreality of the object is the construction of that which is not, and this is interdependent own-being. The structure has no substance because it is only a series of changing relations among the members of a set of elements according to one or more codes. The construction of that which is not, allows emptiness to be known: the Being of non-being = the Real.

Afflicted and Clear Emptiness

The Real and emptiness are forms of jouis-'Sense', as forms of the Third jouissance of meaning. At this juncture, the term meaning is the best among the three terms that could be used within Lacanian theory (meaning, signification, and significance [*signifiance*]). Jouissance, the Real, and emptiness are all related yet independent concepts that share the quality of being beyond concepts or being the 'no concept', or a signifier without a signified.

The 'no concept' or Name is the clear screen/state in which all things exist in their emptiness. The clear screen/state points to a form of energy and mind (jouissance) that Freud described in his Metapsychology. The clear screen that both protected Joyce from madness and revealed the structure of madness, is the *Sinthome*, or the NoF coming from the Real. The clear screen 'screens' as the word indicates and afforded Joyce protection from traditional beliefs, and his own demons and delusions, that could not stick to the screen. Such protection is associated with the Pcpt-Cs. system rather than the Pcs-Pcpt system. The Pcpt.-Cs. system differs from the conditioned consciousness in the Pcs.Pcpt system or the Pcs.Pcpt.-Cs system.

Cognition includes a form of the mind and reason that goes beyond concepts and beyond itself. Nous in Aristotle is one of the four types of human reason that he defined. Nous can be conceived as the layer of the Mind/reason that is a clear sheet/screen of awareness without a subject or object. Now we can add Nous to the various definitions of the clear screen/state: NoF from the Real; *sinthome*; fourth ring; null set; awareness; *sujet san substance*; emptiness; non-thinking; non-knowing; an intention without an object.

Since the clear screen does not keep any registrations or inscriptions of its own, one can say that there is a layer of the mind where cognitions temporarily end. At the same time the clear state of mind continuously assigns cognitions an element of non-existence.

Cognition is equivalent to inscription, representation, signifier, mark, etc., and the various Codes that organize the battery of elements and the sense of reality. Cognitions function according to interdependent symbolic representations but generate no obstruction to access the Real. The Real reveals the non-being of signifiers, or how they exist by not existing, and at the same time the Imaginary has its own way of using the battery of signifiers, as images, to represent/supplant the Real.

For cognitivism, the guiding model is the digital computer. A computation is an operation performed on symbols for purposes of calculation. Cognitivism ignores the difference between a human mental representation and how a computer uses and manipulates symbols outside the human dimension of Sense, desire, intentionality, jouissance, and outside awareness. Although Nous, as a form of human reason, may not have a subject or an object, this still differs from the absence of human sense found within digital computers.

In addition, in contrast to a computer, a human symbol/signifier is a signifier of desire as a human intention. Husserl conceived of the *noema* as intentionality without linguistic meaning or what Lacan would call a pure desire. The meaning here is in the Real of jouissance and this form of experience is something that computers are not capable of having. Meaning in the Real is when meaning is outside or not inside the signifier: the place of meaning is occupied by jouissance as an experience outside meaning.

The Real as distinct from (virtual) reality is a human dimension of experience that at the same time goes beyond the subject-object concepts that characterize human experience. It is out of the undetermined Real within the knot that new signifiers can emerge for the subject. Computers are not capable of doing anything other than follow a program. A computer by itself (without a human being) is not capable of inventing anything new without first being given a program or Code by a human being.

The human screen differs from a computer screen because the clear screen is a part of the Pcpt.-Cs. system as a dimension of the human mind that also includes a form of awareness beyond consciousness. Because the clear screen does not have content of its own or is not determined by the content of the signifiers that pass through it, the clear screen also corresponds to a stable reservoir of base level potential energy and the experience of clarity, lucidity of mind, and a state of non-affliction or '*non-a-fiction*'.

Wittingly or unwittingly, clarity of mind and breathing is what we say yes to on a regular basis even if we don't believe in assenting or saying yes to the NoF, and whether we believe the NoF is a legitimate concept or not.

That clarity of Mind can be assented to, is something almost uncontroversial perhaps, like the clarity of gold, water, and space.

Clarity seeks the attainment of a pure pair of constructed and uncompounded constructions. Clarity is to be illumined about ignorance and the power of opposites or opposite charges to attract or repel one another, whether between electrical charges, ideas, or human beings. Speaking beings cannot avoid raising specks of dust and creating minor forms of disturbance, but a mishandling of opposites generates unnecessary disturbances and obfuscations.

The way out from a conflict between two opposite points of view is not to find a third position that 'sublates' (to use a happy Hegelian term) the prior two, because the third or the 'sin-thesis' itself become a new thesis opposed by an antithesis, and so on and so forth. The chain is broken, and we pluck and raise the living flower (as Buddha and Marx would have it) when the opposition is perceived inside or within the subject rather than as an external imposition coming from the Other. Oppositions are immanent to the subject. To effectively handle the disturbance produced between opposing subjects/arguments a subject must first listen to the Other as the discourse of their own unconscious, before they know how to respond to an opposing argument stated by another subject.

Assenting to clarity and non-affliction can only function as medicine and alleviation if at the same time clarity and lucidity do not reject cogitations because cogitations and Nous provide the structure that is not/naught. Cogitation on one side, and clarity and non-thought on the other, is <u>like</u> particle and wave, energy and matter. Clarity is like wave and energy and cogitation is like particle and matter.

The emptiness of the non-rejection of cognitions is for the sake of clearing the own-being and transmission of a lineage. Psychoanalysis is a lineage that by many accounts needs to place its own house and being in order.

There are two ways for analysts to comprise reality together:

1. By means of signs/signifiers that apprehend the world of the senses and human relationships;
2. By means of Naming that apprehends to worlds of concepts and principles.

So long as we remain aware that constructions (being constructions of what it is not) are only interdependent phenomena, then constructions do allow emptiness or the Real to be known. Constructions are not for mainly two reasons: first, because constructions are typically virtual (on paper) or arise first in the imagination; and second, because of the nature of structural interdependence. All the elements in a structure exist as a function of the relation with other elements. In themselves and by themselves each element is empty of the definitions given by the Code. Since each element is empty while it functions in relationship to the other elements of the structure, one can say that the structure is foundationally empty or Real. The sub-atomic structure of matter itself is empty given the amount of empty space that exists between particles.

Awareness, as previously defined, is not to be confused with the existence or non-existence of objects. Consciousness is always consciousness of something or is conditioned by an object, but awareness has neither subject nor object.

References

Beck, A. T. (1967). *The Diagnosis and Management of Depression*. Philadelphia: University of Pennsylvania Press.

Freud, A. (1936 [1992]). *The Ego and the Mechanisms of Defence*. London: Karnac.

Lacan, J. (1956 [2006]). *Ecrits*. The First Complete Edition in English (B. Fink, Trans.). Seminar on the Purloined Letter (pp. 6–48). First published in French in 1966. New York: Norton and Norton.

Lacan, J. (1971a). *El Seminario de Jacques Lacan. Libro 19...o peor*. Buenos Aires: Paidos.

Lacan, J. (1971b). *...ou pire. Seminar XIX* (C. Gallagher, Trans.). Unpublished. www.lacaninireland.com. Accessed 29 Aug 2017.

Lacan, J. (1971c). *The Seminar of Jacques Lacan XVIII: On a Discourse That Might Not Be a Semblance* (C. Gallagher, Trans.). London: Karnac.

9

The Other Psychoanalysis and the Other in Psychoanalysis

In Seminar XVII Lacan (1969–1970) speaks of the three different discourses that interact with the discourse of the analyst: university, hysteric/clinical, and the discourse of the master or of government.

Lacan distinguishes between discourse and speech and calls his teaching a discourse that approaches Freud from the Other side or the theoretical underside of psychoanalytic practice. Discourse or theory is a structure that exceeds the use of words or speech. Psychoanalysis needs both a discourse (the discourse of the analyst) and the use of speech in the practice of analysis. Discourse refers to a structure and to a social link and practice that also constitutes a form of *savoir* or knowing from experience that is produced in the analytic situation. Freud and Lacan are authors who wrote outside the university but have become a source of ideas to produce interpretation and the practice of science within the university.

In this chapter I want to explore the notion of the Other psychoanalysis in relationship to Lacanian psychoanalysis. The Other psychoanalysis does not refer to the theoretical or academic Other side of psychoanalysis (as the title of Lacan's Seminar XVII has been translated) but to another influential orientation within psychoanalysis: object

R. Moncayo, *Knowing, Not-Knowing, and Jouissance*, The Palgrave Lacan Series,
https://doi.org/10.1007/978-3-319-94003-8_9

relations. I will use the work of Winnicott as representative of this orientation although Bion could have been used just as well.

Winnicott's work is less academic and more phenomenological, although not without theory, and stays grounded in the clinical practice of analysis. The object relations school does not have a concept of the Other that Lacan borrowed from philosopy (specifically from Hegel—a philosopher that the English were not fond off), and instead expands the concept of the object found in Freud. Winnicott is critical of arm chair philosophers and at times even seems self-conscious of the simplicity of his theory as if, perhaps, he could be accused of being too simplistic by Freud himself (if he were alive). Nonetheless, his work is important for psychoanalysis and it would not be too far-fetched to say that the object relations and Lacanian schools represent the future of psychoanalysis.

In contrast to Klein (2017), and Freud, Winnicott (1963) lends more importance to what he calls the maturational environment and the actual parent-child relationship than to the focus on unconscious fantasy found in Freud and Klein. Lacan for his part wanted to return to Freud but in the end developed a new theory for psychoanalysis however grounded in Freudian theory it may be (or not). Winnicott also knew about Lacan and his theory of the mirror stage that would have been relevant to his work with children, but he chose to ignore Lacan's work and not get involved in the IPA's exclusion of Lacan (a form of complicity, therefore).

Winnicott emphasizes a distinction between subjective objects and objective objects, and thus the term object relations no longer mean unconscious relations among unconscious part objects (*objet a* and the phallus in Lacan). Objects now refer to whole objects and actual subjects or persons in the world. This distinction was ambiguous in Freud although when talking about love, for example, in "*Drives and their Vicissitudes*" (1915), he associated love to the ego and whole object relations. In the US object relations is associated with a blend of ego psychology, object relations, and interpersonal or relational psychoanalysis. Invariably, the focus on the external environment and whole object or interpersonal relations leads away from the focus on the Unconscious and unconscious fantasy, and their relationships to the concept of drive in Lacan and instincts as understood in biology and Darwinian theory, which has increasingly become the theory for biological science.

Of course, Freud thought instinct in humans appears as drives constituted within symbolic and cultural orders. North American 'cultural' psychoanalysis' lack of understanding of this point often leads them to make of Freud's alleged biologism of instinct a straw man that they can attack while misunderstanding or ignoring Lacanian or European psychoanalysis that has developed well beyond this point (Mitchell, 2000).

Lacan denounced the deviations from Freud's theory even though the language of ego and whole object relations was initiated by Freud himself. The focus on the external environment points to the biological environment and not necessarily to the cultural environment. Biological adaptation to the environment is a Darwinian concept that applies to living biological systems. The fact that one is focused on the environment instead of the so-called intrapsychic world does not mean that we have left the biological realm. Conversely, if one focuses on the intrapsychic world it does not mean we have left the cultural world either.

What does Winnicott's maturational environment mean beyond Freud's notion of external reality or world? The mother is the maturational environment for an infant. More than that, it is not only a question of maternal preoccupation or care giving because what is important, according to Lacanian theory, is to be the object of the mother's desire or *objet a* cause of desire. Privation is considered by Winnicott as a negative and damaging influence on the maternal environment. But apparently being a Kleinian, or because of not being a Kleinian, he does not understand the loss or separation from the breast (weaning) as a form of necessary privation. The latter is the negative influence of the environment and of the father but that is necessary for the child to become a subject in culture.

The same goes for frustration and symbolic castration. If we only understand these as injuring in a negative sense, then we may give off the unrealistic impression that we can have an ideal environment without privation, frustration, and castration. Since this is an impossibility because these negatives are also positive for subjectivity, we miss out on their positive impact, and due to the inevitability of the pain produced by them, we set up higher and higher ideals of non-traumatic environments that if only we could build them right and perfect them, then the absence of pathology would be possible. To be fair to Winnicott, when he speaks of privation he may be speaking not of the necessary absence of the breast (the bad breast) but of the failure or unreliability of the good breast to show up and provide at all.

The difference here is a consequence of the two theories (Lacan's and Winnicott's) being differentially placed with respect to the paternal/parental metaphor. Freud and Lacan have been accused of being father-centred while Klein, Bion, and Winnicott are mother-centred. There is no father function in any of them. The mother is present in Lacan as one of the two elements of the paternal metaphor: $\frac{NoF}{\textit{Desire of the Mother}}$. In fact, the equation works the same way if you place either term as numerator or denominator. If the mother is on top, then the signified for the signifier of the mother's desire is the NoF. If the father is on top the signified for the NoF is the object of the mother's desire. Whether one is on top and the other is not, what matters is that neither can exist without the other. The desire of the mother needs the NoF to appear as a signifier, and the NoF does not have meaning without the enigma of the mother's desire.

With this clarification of terms in mind, let us examine the depth of Winnicott's theories more closely. In his paper on "Communicating and Not Communicating Leading to a Study of Certain Opposites (1963)", he stakes out a twofold claim for an isolated individual on the one hand, and a capacity for object relatedness, on the other. The individual is "a non-communicating self, or the personal core of the self that is a true isolate." Non-communication also means quietude and stillness.

The individual's non-communicating self, or the personal core of the self that is a true isolate, does not simply represent a failure in object relatedness, unless the isolation is a rejection of relating and communicating due to a failure of the facilitating environment. For Winnicott (1963) the primary narcissism associated with what he calls the isolate individual is not a narcissistic defence against relating but rather the positive aspects of the fusion with the mother that leads to baby talk, lalangue, and the joy of speech.

> When her reliability dominates the scene the infant could be said to communicate simply by going on being, and by going on developing according to personal processes of maturation, but this scarcely deserves the epithet communication. (p. 188)

Thanks to the secure environment-mother, the child can be alone in the presence of the mother and develop a subjectivity where his/her experience could be private. Fantasy life and waking reverie would be an example of this. This aspect is found in adults in the capacity to keep thoughts private and only communicate those that are socially acceptable or that can be communicated with language. One can argue that this is associated with the normative persona that many would consider an imaginary form of false self and cogito, but Winniccott only reserves the category of the false self to a false adaptation to a non-facilitating environment. The facilitating environment is the mother that desires or loves the child, in addition to providing necessary care-giving. This allows for the child to have an isolate self that can chose to communicate or not communicate. The child communicates with the facilitating mother and adapts to her requests and care giving.

In Lacanian theory, and in accordance with primary narcissism, there is a pre-subject prior to a subject-object differentiation, but the subject of the Real and what Lacan (1971–1972) calls the subject "All-alone" is a result of a realization of the lack of sexual rapport between the sexes. And as I have explained elsewhere (Moncayo, 2017), the lack of rapport between the sexes does not necessarily mean that this lack translates to an absence of relationships or sexual activity in the descriptive or phenomenological sense.

However, the relationship with the mother is one of sameness and unconditional love in the sense that the child is loved even if they don't know how to speak, cannot walk well, or has no motor coordination and throws objects around. This will change with maturity where the so-called adaptation to the environment will have many more rules and expectations associated with it. These include hygiene, sleep schedules, chores, homework, and play. This is where the function of the father becomes more important in establishing the ego ideal as the agency that regulates the ideals that dictate what should be done, and the super ego that dictates what should not be done. In preparation for the symbolic father, the symbolic mother also provides ego-support to the child in the form of providing support rooted in the earlier relationship but now applied to support the child's acquisition of hygiene, sleep schedule, chores, homework, and play. The child can withdraw from communicating with the mother and not lose her love because the child is applying himself/herself to a task designated by the mother.

But why is there a need for rules that compel the ego to relate to culture in ways that may not seem facilitating to the ego? The answer comes from the relationship to the object mother. Fantasies are linked to the love and hate of the object mother. Fantasies grow in the transitional or potential space (to use Winnicott's terms) provided by a subjective object that for the subject seems to afford a more real form of experience.

Paradoxically for Winnicott (2011) object relatedness or relation refers to the fantasy object or subjective object. The objective object comes with what he calls object usage. The fantasy object is related to the object mother or the mother as an object of fantasy.

> "Object-relating is an experience of the subject that can be described in terms of the subject as an isolate."[...] When I speak of the use of an object, however, I take object-relating for granted, and add new features that involve the nature and the behaviour of the object. For instance, the object, if it is to be used, must necessarily be real in the sense of being part of shared reality, not a bundle of projections. (p. 254)

Object usage refers to the concept of objective object. However, in what he called object relation to the fantasy object there already existed a relation to the actions of the object given that the mother communicates to the child that the child is the object of her fantasy. The objective object is never a thing-in-itself as Winnicott says because he confuses the symbolic nature of the other as an objective object with the Real nature of the object as a thing or no-thing independent from the symbolic other (objective object) and the object of fantasy.

In other words, Winnicott's theory misses the concept of the other/ Other to describe the objective object as well as the nature of the Real rather than reality. For Lacanians, the only whole object is the image of the body which is other to the ego even if it is its own image. The total image of the other is predicated first on the total image of the ideal ego (body image) that in turn is predicated on the desire of the Other that establishes a causal series or a chain of dependent origination. In addition, the concept of the intersubjective other depends on the concept of the big Other or the Other of culture. Lacan brings these concepts together by speaking of the partial fantasy object as small *objet a*; the neighbour, sibling, or alter ego is the small other; and the Other is the Other of Culture and the battery of signifiers. *Objet a* is derived from the *a* for autre (other) in French.

In Lacan the transition from *objet a* or fantasy object to the objective object of external reality and society is achieved via the ideal ego, the alter ego, and the Other. The transition requires symbolic castration and the loss of the object and its consequent symbolization. But Winnicott means something else when speaking of the transition to object usage. For Winnicott an analyst must carry an analysand from object relation to object usage and he adds the twist that in object usage the object is destroyed and, paradoxically, the object survives the destruction. The child says then to the destroyed object that survived the destruction: "I destroyed you, I love you" (the reverse of Lacan's [1964] "I love you, I mutilate you" referring to the *objet a*). Winnicott's thesis has the surprising effect of proposing that objectivity or the objective object is discovered or created through its destruction. Of course, that this is a development of the Klein's (1940) depressive position where the child mourns the destruction of the good breast alongside the destruction of the bad breast. The child fantasizes that the good breast has been destroyed by the attacks on the bad object.

In Lacanian theory, the symbol that provides an objective reference represents the death of the object, so this would be consistent with the destruction of the object, except that in the history of the species what survives the death of the object (the dead bull/cow) is the unary trace as the beginning of number and the signifier. The symbol survives the death of the object within a system of substitutive/methaphoric links to other signifiers and between signifiers. There are links between ideas/signifiers, and also between love and hate (Bion, 1962). The destruction of the object also parallels the lack of rapport between the sexes resulting from the friction between the object of fantasy (*objet a*) and the body/mind of the intersubjective other. Both parties to a relationship have to survive each other.

The subject accesses the other/Other, when the fantasy object as an omnipotent object is destroyed by the subject in relationship to the Other. Either the analysand 'kills' the analyst and the analyst survives or, vice versa, in a symbolic formulation, the analytical function 'kills' or symbolically castrates the analysand and a new subject emerges. The analyst is already a lacking symbolic other through the power of their own unconscious. Such lack/luck manifests through the analyst's use of authority as a suspended function. In the void represented by the analyst's silence, and the analyst occupying the place of the absence of the object and the lack in the Other, fantasies emerge to respond to the question: what does the Other want from me? Once the subject is no longer fooled by the fantasy, then the other can be used as Other or signifier as well as object of fantasy.

What is unique about Winnicott is that he says that the price paid to access the other/Other is not the symbolic castration of the subject but the acceptance of the destruction of the fantasy object in relationship to the Other. The Other is no longer a fantasy object because the fantasy object has fallen to waste and become expendable. The destruction of the object in this sense does not only apply to the aggressiveness towards the object because the analyst, for example, must fall from the position of the *objet a* and must become expendable for there to be a logical end to the analysis. But according to Winnicott, this is not only an outcome of how the analyst abandons the position of the subject supposed to know in the transference. Nevertheless, for all practical purposes, the fall of idealization love may share some similarities with what Winnicott calls the destruction of the object.

In Lacanian analysis, hate in the transference, or the de-supposition of the Other as the subject supposed to know, is not the same as the analyst in Lacanian analysis no longer occupying the position of the subject supposed to know. When this happens, unconscious knowing is located on the side of the unconscious of the analysand. The Lacanian view represents a working through the love transference, but Winnicott's involves the working through the negative transference. Lacanians don't recommend working through the negative transference ("A negative transference…must be dispensed with as soon as possible". Verhaegue, 2001, p. 38), although both approaches end up in the place where the object has been used for the purpose of realizing the subject's desire (the preservation of the love of the object, in the case of Winiccott, or that the object lives in the subject's own desire or Ucs., in the case of Lacan).

Since at the end of Lacanian analysis, the analyst must become dispensable, or the analysand may be said to have had enough of the analyst, it can be argued that in a Lacanian analysis, the analysis ends thanks to the negative transference despite the negative transference not having been interpreted in the course of the analysis. Negative transference refers here to the antipathy (hate would be too strong of a word in this context) that may arise associated with the difficult work with unconscious lack and symbolic castration. Such antipathy (Winnicott uses the word hate for this phenomenon) would be Symbolic (reality) in this case, although the Symbolic would also lead to an opening towards the Lacanian Real. Lacan says the Real is an obstacle and to this extent the Real would also be engaged in symbolic antipathy. In any case such understanding of the negative transference as a catalyst for the end of analysis needs to be differentiated from the ordinary conception of the negative transference defined by Lacan as de-supposing the analyst as 'subject supposed to know': "What do you know, or you are wrong about me, and this analysis is not helping, etc."

In Seminar XX (Section VIII on knowledge and truth) Lacan (1972–1973) speaks of what he calls hateloving (*L'hainamoration*) and argues that knowledge about love always gives rise to hate as its regular underside. Converting love into knowledge gives rise to hate and this is something linked to symbolic knowledge that does not amount to an imaginary form of hatred associated with fantasies and death wishes. Instead love without knowledge or when the latter remains unknown (unknown-knowing), does not give rise to hate. Not interpreting (to be differentiated from its analysis in the speech of the analysand) the love transference would also help keep this form of hate at bay. Knowledge in this context can be defined as connaissance or cognizing/discriminating rather than as *savoir*. *Savoir* is a form of knowing that does not exist ('ex-sists') or is consistent with non-knowing and Nous as a basis for analytical listening. In this definition, *savoir* about love would either not give rise to hate or help contain love's inevitable pair-wise companion.

The attribution of knowledge to the analyst in the transference is experienced as symbolic castration, since the analyst presumably is the one that knows about lack. "The Other that knows about love hates me, and I hate what I perceive that the Other knows about love." Cephalic connaissance (cognition) must be symbolically castrated in order to access *savoir* in the Real of being. The knowledge in the Other, perceived as hate, must be accepted, and the hate for the knowledge in and of the Other will eventually subside. Herein lies the question that Winnicott raises with regards to so-called objective hate that must be survived.

Lacan had to survive the jealousy, envy, and negative transferences within his own school that at some point led him to dissolve it. For Winnicott, the first impulse and relationship to the object is destructive rather than libidinal. It all depends on the definition of the object that we are speaking about: the object involved in object usage and/or the object of the fantasy. It is easier to understand the relation to the external world and the objective object as based on hate and fear. In this both Freud and Klein agreed but for different reasons. For Freud, external reality was unpleasant because of the frustrations, disappointments, and castrations involved in the interaction with the father, culture, and surviving in the social world. For Klein, the object world is unpleasant because of the frustrations and aggression associated with the bad breast. Obviously the two views are not necessarily opposed, and in fact Lacanian theory resolves the conflict between the two positions. Privation, frustration, and castration, involve different zones and phases/faces of development. Finally, all would agree that the relationship to the fantasy object is based on love and desire.

Winnicott argues that aggressiveness and the survival of the object is involved in the construction of the external world. To use the analyst as a symbolic Other, the analyst must allow and survive the analysand's attack more than interpret. Winnicott thinks that the fantasy object is always being destroyed. In the end, we come back to the idea that it is the fantasy object that is destroyed but not the Other. However, the fantasy object can never be completely annihilated because otherwise there will be no desire without fantasy. What is possible is not to be fooled by the fantasy or confuse the fantasy object for the other or the usage of the object.

References

Bion, W. (1962 [2004]). *Learning from Experience*. Oxford: Rowman & Littlefield.

Freud, S. (1915). *Instincts and Their Vicissitudes*. SE, 14, 111–140.

Klein, M. (1940 [1975]). Mourning and Its Relation to Manic-Depressive States. In *Love, Guilt and Reparation and Other Works 1921–1945* (The Writings of Melanie Klein, Vol. 1). New York: The Free Press.

Klein, M. (1975 [2017]). *The Collected Works of Melanie Klein*. London: Karnac.

Lacan, J. (1964 [1981]). *The Four Fundamental Concepts of Psychoanalysis*. New York: Norton.

Lacan, J. (1969–1970 [2007]). *The Seminar of Jacques Lacan: Book XVII: The Other Side of Psychoanalysis*. London: Routledge.

Lacan, J. (1971–1972). *...ou pire. Seminar XIX*. (C. Gallagher, Trans.). Unpublished. www.lacaninireland.com. Accessed 29 Aug 2017.

Lacan, J. (1998 [1972–1973]). *The Seminar of Jacques Lacan XX: On Feminine Sexuality or the Limits of Love and Knowledge*. New York: Norton.

Mitchell, S. (2000). *Relationality. From Attachment to Intersubjectivity*. New Jersey: The Analytic Press.

Moncayo, R. (2017). *Lalangue, Sinthome, Jouissance, and Nomination. A Reading Companion and Commentary on Lacan's Seminar XXIII on the Sinthome*. London: Karnac.

Verhague, P. (2001). *Beyond Gender. From Subject to Drive*. New York: Other Press.

Winnicott, D. (1963 [2011]). Communicating and Not Communicating Leading to a Study of Certain Opposites. In L. Coldwell & A. Joyce (Eds.), *Reading Winnicott*. London: Routledge.

Winnicott, D. (2011). *Reading Winnicott*, L. Coldwell & A. Joyce (Eds.). London: Routledge.

10

Standard and Non-Standard Frames for the Practice of Analysis and the Question of Pure and Applied Psychoanalysis

This chapter is geared towards practicing psychoanalysts in private practice. When speaking of private practice, I do not refer to services solely available to the upper classes which is how psychoanalysis was first understood in the US. This was primarily due to the long past association between psychoanalysis and the business-based medical establishment. Private here refers to Freud's belief that psychoanalysis can only thrive in democratic rather than totalitarian societies. It is in the private sector where the subject may find some relief from the family, society, and the state. Both applied and non-standard analysis take different shapes in both private and public/institutional settings. When describing non-standard analyses, this chapter is primarily referring to applied psychoanalysis in a private practice setting. However, it is also possible to apply Lacanian psychoanalysis to a public or institutional setting but this would be a related but different subject than the one presently under consideration. In an analytical school, both the personal and control analysis of an analyst in formation takes place in private practice.

I would like to first introduce and define some of the basic terms I will be using in this chapter. Let's start with defining pure and applied psychoanalysis. Pure psychoanalysis refers to psychical or mental phenomena

R. Moncayo, *Knowing, Not-Knowing, and Jouissance*, The Palgrave Lacan Series,
https://doi.org/10.1007/978-3-319-94003-8_10

and interventions or practices associated with and only with psychoanalysis in a strict sense. The speech or mental phenomena addressed by pure psychoanalysis refers to unconscious material and true speech regarding desire rather than to conscious narratives or stories about everyday things, although desire can also be embedded in the latter.

In addition, pure can also refer to interventions that are justified by theoretical criteria and not solely by practical rules. However, pure psychoanalysis should not be construed as only theoretical or academic since it also refers to the derivation of the theory from the unconscious signifying chain. Applied psychoanalysis refers to the application of psychoanalysis to clinical practice and treatment in general but more specifically it refers to the alleviation of symptoms and mental or emotional suffering (Miller, 2015). These two categories are also intimately related to the next set of basic categories: the standard and the non-standard analysis or treatment.

Typically people think of the standard or classical treatment and pure psychoanalysis as being the same, but this is not necessarily the case. Pure psychoanalysis is defined by the material or mental and emotional phenomena disclosed and worked on during the treatment. The standard analysis refers to the setting, the furniture and tools or technology used, and the frequency and length of both sessions and treatments. The non-standard treatment may vary with respect to the frame (variable length and frequency of sessions and treatment) but works on similar material and may achieve the same results as pure psychoanalysis, a classical analysis, and applied psychoanalysis (symptom improvement or resolution). Conversely, the standard analysis may work on material that may not be consistent with pure psychoanalysis and achieve or not the results expected from applied psychoanalysis.

The third set of categories refers to the distinction between psychoanalysis and psychotherapy. On the one hand, psychotherapy refers to the definition of applied psychoanalysis and to the conception of psychoanalysis as a method of clinical treatment. Psychoanalysis is a form of psychotherapeutic treatment. On the other hand, psychotherapy can be differentiated from psychoanalysis, as a sub-category of psychoanalysis in the case of psychoanalytic psychotherapy, or as an alternative to psychoanalysis in the case of treatments that have been developed after psychoanalysis and against psychoanalysis.

'Psychoanalysis' or 'Freudian psychoanalysis' became taboo within the clinic of evidence-based practices. There are many reasons for this being the case despite the fact that a close cousin of psychoanalysis, psychodynamic psychotherapy, has been shown to be efficacious in evidence-based-controlled studies (Schedler, 2010). Meta-analysis by Leichsenring, F. and Rabung, S. (2008/2009) proved that Long Term Psychodynamic Psychotherapy (LTPP) showed significantly higher outcomes in overall effectiveness, target problems, and personality functioning than shorter forms of psychotherapy. It also showed that LTPP patients with complex mental disorders on average were better off than 96% of the patients in the comparison groups ($P=0.002$). Thus, within the psychodynamic field widely construed, there are many who consider psychodynamic psychotherapy a more efficient treatment than psychoanalysis.

However, despite the evidence LTPP is not a widely used form of psychotherapy. If it is practiced, it is mostly in the private sector of health care as opposed to Cognitive Behavioral Therapy (CBT) and Dialectical Behavioral Therapy (DBT) that are practiced widely in mental health clinics, community clinics, academic centers, and university hospitals, where the cost of long term treatment may be considered prohibitive.

When it comes to psychoanalysis the situation is even worse and below we will discuss how psychoanalysis has had a big role to play in this being the case. There seems to be an interesting dissemination bias that considers psychoanalysis as an outdated form of treatment that is rarely used mostly because of its lack of efficacy. This conviction is being repeated like a gospel not only between health care professionals, but also between health care policy makers and researchers.

There are a number of studies that prove the contrary. For example a study performed by Busch, Milrod, and Sandberg (2013) not only demonstrated the efficacy of psychoanalytic treatment for panic disorder but also provided guidelines on ways psychoanalysis could be introduced into the era of evidence-based medicine. There is also empirical evidence that psychoanalysis, as a long-term psychotherapeutic treatment, produces more robust results and outcomes over time. The relapse rates of short-term treatments such as CBT or medications tend to increase over time while the after termination results of psychoanalysis indicate that patients get better over time and the analysis tends to continue producing effects post-termination. The evidence for these results comes from controlled studies and not only from consumer reports studies of outcome (Levy, Ablon, & Kächele, 2011).

Since its inception, psychoanalysis has not relied on statistical sampling methods and control groups but has operated according to the single clinical case study method as a point of articulation between theory and clinical practice. In addition, there is a practical problem in presenting the empirical evidence revealed in the practice of psychoanalysis as a treatment method.

The problem is social, ethical, and legal in nature. People often complain that Lacan never spoke about cases and this is contrasted to Freud's presentation of famous case histories. However, despite Freud's attempts to disguise and protect the identity of his patients, one by one historians eventually revealed the identities of most if not all his analysands. Lacan did not even try to speak about his patients because many of them were in the audience during his seminars and had he talked about them he could not possibly have kept their life and identity private. Nowadays extensive psychoanalytic case histories cannot be published without written consent from the patients. Statistically-based studies using experimental and control groups also require prior consent but the material reported in these studies differs greatly from the unconscious material disclosed in analytical sessions. The latter typically contains much more sensitive and confidential information.

Psychologists or psychiatrists who do empirical research rarely engage the kind of material that analysands speak to their analyst during the course of an analysis, so their data invariably remains within the normal socially acceptable narrative that people could share about themselves with anyone. In addition, empirically based theories are also constructed on the basis of surface constructs that match the conscious narratives and concerns of people.

Then measures are constructed on the basis of such constructs where the questions asked from research subjects are entirely based on the conscious narratives of patients. Conscious narratives and words can be analysed and counted in various ways and there have been empirical studies doing precisely this (Pennebaker, 1995, 1997). However, these studies are limited to disclosures of traumatic experiences, or to such things as determining hidden motivations in the texts written by terrorists or determining a subject's health status by analyzing their use of causal words or personal pronouns.

Finally, the empirical subjects used in empirical or evidence-based behavioral practice (EBP) are often university students that differ greatly from the populations seen in clinical practice. Thus, clinical experience may be wider than the evidence produced in statistical research and not only vice versa. What works in the clinic may not be proven by controlled studies, and what is proven efficient in academic studies, may not work in the clinic. Most university researchers are not clinicians, as well as vice versa. In fact, when EBP is used in the clinic, the rates of clinical effectiveness are not greater than that of clinicians not using EBP. The two aspects of clinical experience and the singularity of each subject are the hallmarks of the psychoanalytic observational and scientific method since Freud.

Theory and practice do not form two complementary pieces of a whole or directly translate or correspond with one another. There is no bi-univocal one-to-one correspondence between theory and practice. Either one or the other tends to be excluded in the process. Either an excess of theory eclipses the possibility of thinking about patients and interventions, or focusing on patients and interventions makes for a more restricted theory. Theory and practice cannot be substituted for one another without a loss of truth. The correspondence between theory and practice is artificial or made up. The substitution of theory for practice or practice for theory leads to a reduplication of the field of truth. Where there was one truth now there are two.

The reason for this being the case, according to Lacanian theory, is that truth can only be half-said and, therefore, there is always a truth that remains unsaid interacting with a relative truth that has been said. These two truths are neither one nor two. What ever you say, in the relative 'fictional' side of truth, always has another side not being said, and the trick is to leave it unsaid, or say it in a saying rather than a statement, to avoid being falsely mislead by the promise of another substitution that also will not be "It" or will not be the side of truth that is in the Real.

When the theory, for example, speaks of a repressive and a repressed force, in the clinic these concepts are replaced by the technical concepts of process and content. Process points to defenses at work in speech and relationships while content refers to the nature of the material being spoken about. Words substitute other words but we are not necessarily closer to the referential empirical objects that the words represent.

According to psychoanalysis mental objects are often missing or unconscious. But this so-called unconscious can either not exist, and be a mere supposition without empirical support, or it may exist but it is only known through representations. The Unconscious is repressed or hidden from perception but nonetheless produces effects and determines real phenomena and experience. In addition, the Unconscious may represent something that is beyond language or categorical description of any kind (theoretical or practical). What is Real in the Lacanian sense may always differ from the reality of the object as defined within logical, semantic, or theoretical constructs.

The Real in Lacan is a dimension of experience that lies beyond words or images although an "interior" aspect of it can manifest in poetic language, the creative imagination, jouissance, and topology. The Real unconscious is to be distinguished from the repressed unconscious because the Real unconscious has nothing repressed in it (images or words) but is an aspect of experience that is beyond representation. Lacan makes a clear differentiation between the Real and his two other registers: Imaginary and Symbolic. However, at the same time he claims that his mathemes (symbolic mathematical formulas that are not arithmetical in nature) help us in approaching the Real. In Badiou and Roudinesco's (2014) words:

> the Real of the subject is unsymbolizable. As a result, Lacan goes as far as possible in formalization in order to experience a fundamental impasse. At some point, the integral formalization should break down because it no longer has a hold on the very thing it is trying to grasp. This is the moment when we touch on the real point of the subject. (p. 50)

A good way to conceptualize the conundrum of the Real is to use the example of some of the findings of modern physics. Take, for example, the uncertainty principle formulated by Heisenberg. Heisenberg showed that position and velocity cannot both be measured at the same time.

Any attempt to measure precisely the velocity of a subatomic particle, such as an electron, will alter its course in such an unpredictable way that renders the results invalid.

The impossibility of the measurement is closely related to the connection between particles and waves in the subatomic realm and it has nothing to do with lack of equipment or flaws in observation techniques. When waves are measured they become particles and lose their superposition or the ability to manifest in more than one place at a time. Einstein had trouble accepting the results of quantum theory and commented by stating that "matter must have a separate reality independent of the measurements. That is, an electron has spin, location and so forth even when it is not being measured. I like to think that the moon is there even if I am not looking at it" (cited by O'Conner, 1999, p. 41). But perhaps the independent reality of the particle is the wave, not the particle itself. What the moon itself is in the Real without the observation or the finger pointing at it we cannot say for a fact.

It is true that the moon is there even when we are not looking at it, however, we should not mistake the moon with our finger pointing at it. In other words reality is not the Real. On the other hand, we would not know anything of it without the observation or the finger pointing at it. Thus the Real is known through what is Real within the Symbolic. The wave is also the particle.

We also have to accept that a theoretical discussion will not immediately translate into an intervention with a patient. To understand this point we must first understand the different types of rationality involved in a scientific endeavor. For Aristotle (1907) there were four types of rationality: Nous, episteme, techne, and practical reason (Moncayo, 2017). Nous represents the relationship between knowing and doubt, or knowing and non-knowing as a source of knowing (I only know that I don't know). In addition, nous represents the contemplation of the first principles. Episteme is how we think about valid knowledge and the relationships between theory and practice or theory and method, etc. Techne is method or experiment, and technology (telescope, phone, internet, etc.). Finally, practical reason refers to ethics, how we think about ethics (of desire or morality), to professional practices, but more fundamentally practical reason also refers to the question of choice, and free will or undeterminism versus determinism.

Free will refers to what we make out of what we are made of. Free will does not deny the existence of a determinate structure especially in matter, but does refer to the fact that the elements or atoms of a structure can be combined in different ways with different results. The elements themselves are Real or empty in the relative sense that they only exist as a function of their interrelationships. However, the Real although empty of concept and definition, does constitute a dimension of experience that is differentially manifest within sense experience (Moncayo & Romanowicz, 2015).

The question whether method, therapeutic or otherwise, can translate into valid theory or whether theory translates into method or techne is an epistemological question. As already stated, for the Greeks the first principles emanate from *Nous* and it is this type of reason or faculty of mind that theoretical discussions strengthen and inspire at the time of their occurrence. Nous is a term for the faculty of the human mind which is necessary for understanding what is true or real.

The phenomena that we study contribute to an awareness that remains independent and undefined by the content of what is learned or who is doing the learning. Aristotle (De Anima, Book III) referred to it as separate, and as being without attributes and unmixed. As such it constitutes a link between the known and the unknown and even between the known and that which can never be completely known or defined. In many ways it corresponds to what Freud called the free floating awareness of the analyst without a specific subject or object. This definition of Nous avoids the paradox of referring to an unconscious awareness although Lacan does speak of unknown knowing or "*l'insu qui sait*." When an analyst is in the presence of his/her patient's speech the quality of *Nous* will also be there with the analyst. And although the analyst may not be thinking of the theory, the first principles that matter will also be there for his/her disposition and use.

Finally, when discussing cases, from an ethical/practical point of view the clinician/analyst will have to continue to disguise and modify clinical material in order to say the truth about truth. It is important to remember that the challenge that we are facing is not only a question of protecting patients' privacy but also the impossibility to describe, measure, or scale every aspect of psychoanalytic sessions. Even the best, most accurate description of it will not stand for the "real thing." This is why Aristotle's four types of reason cannot be substituted for one another nor remain unrelated. But in order not to fall into the ethical chaos of anything goes, the hierarchy and circularity of mental functions needs to be preserved.

With respect to the circularity and relationship among the different categories of reason an interesting relationship exists between practical reason and *techne*, method, or technique. Practice means that the singular individual has to be directly engaged in a Real practice or specific type of activity rather than simply treated as a number or a constituent of a set, category, or experiment. The treatment method of free association, for example, constitutes ways of unchaining thoughts/feelings or truth from pre-determined chains of thinking, knowledge or prejudice/ideology. The theory or the first principles orient us towards the Real of a practice but do not constitute it or absorb it into the closed circularity of established discourse. This way the theory can change the practice and the practice inform the theory but without either one being reduced to each other. Both the Real of the theory and the Real of the practice have to remain open or unsaturated as well as related to one another.

Hans Steiner (1977) has pointed out that when faced with the question of the scientific status of psychoanalysis, one is bewildered by the array of opinions, both theoretical and research based. Despite a great degree of accumulation of research data showing that psychoanalysis or psychoanalytic psychotherapy is an evidence-based practice, many detractors continue to affirm that psychoanalysis is not an empirical or evidence-based practice that has been objectively tested.

Steiner then asks why is psychoanalysis still an object of controversy despite all the evidence already established? Can this be explained as something more than the simple resistance to the unconscious and to the socially inconvenient truths of desire that need to be quickly brushed aside and hidden under the proverbial carpet? Steiner cites Freud when he stated that although experimental confirmations of psychoanalysis do no harm, psychoanalysis already provides a wealth of reliable observations that are independent from experimental validation. Thus Freud appears to have restricted: "...the process of observation and validation to the analytic situation" (p. 518).

If psychoanalysis is already an empirically derived practice why would it need validation and testing from the outside by people who are not intrinsically involved with the theory and the practice and who have not been analysed? Would this not be a set-up to become a victim of the defenses against unconscious desire and sexuality?

Conversely, does not this make psychoanalysis function like a sect that needs to be validated from the inside only? The answer to this question obviously refers to the need for epistemological critique and the free exercise of critical reason as an indispensable aspect of the scientific method. But it also refers to the need for large samples, random sampling, and quantification, which are also necessary ingredients of scientific research. The problem with this aspect of the scientific method is that the propensities discovered by the repetition of the experiment on many subjects may be an artifice of the assumptions and the 'set-up' of the experiment.

However, the difference between Freud's remarks and the different ways of understanding empiricism and observation are not only a question of the size of the samples and the submission of the data to statistical analysis. The question also refers to the dimensions of reality and the forms of reason being studied and used. There is a dimension of reality (what Lacan calls the Real) that only yields its secrets in the singular case and in an actual practice and not in an experiment. The experiment and finite frequentism in statistics only engage two types of reason (episteme and techne), while Nous and Practical reason are required for the study of the singular case.

This explains why Freud would say that for the singular case the observations produced in the case of a singular analysis and a single session are sufficient. The singular case observation does constitute a test and an evaluation of the theory and the practice although it may not produce the propensities of a random sample and statistical testing. What is important here is not the obstinate or dogmatic insistence on the psychoanalytic method, but the logical argument regarding the import of the singular case for the study of human subjectivity and the existence of different types of rationality. In physics it took only one observation of an eclipse with a telescope to declare true and scientific the entire edifice of Einstein's relativity theory.

On the other hand, psychoanalysts are also responsible for the fate of their profession. For years many health care providers saw them as arrogant and ignorant of the 'real world' realities of public and insurance based mental health services. In addition when we look at the textbooks for trainees we notice that they usually contain a very simplistic look at Freud's ideas, which makes them seem appear silly and outlandish.

After the height of its powers in the 50s, one by one most clinical settings and training hospitals ceased to be psychoanalytic. However, despite the rise of the empirical perspective, in large part this change can be attributed to psychoanalysis itself. Most psychoanalysts under the regulation of the International Psychoanalytic Association (IPS) took a kind of 'all or nothing' or 'take it or leave it' attitude. The new generation of political 'powers that be' and administrators chose the 'nothing' or 'leave it' option resulting in the inevitable decline of psychoanalysis.

There are many reasons for the decline of psychoanalysis but we will only focus on a few. First we will examine reasons internal to psychoanalysis itself that we will associate with a dogmatic epistemological position. This dogmatic position is not only directly associated to the theory but also, and more importantly, to the frame of psychoanalysis. In focusing first on reasons internal to psychoanalysis (for the decline of psychoanalysis) we follow the psychoanalytic ethic of taking personal responsibility for our destiny despite the past and present determinations of the unconscious and of the negative influence of others upon us.

Prior to inventing psychoanalysis (the 'talking cure'), Freud experimented with many treatment methods available at that time such as hypnosis and suggestion. In passing, it is important to note that these methods are still being used today both within and outside psychoanalysis. This is not the place to argue this point but enough is to say that suggestion is an integral part of both research and cognitive behavioral therapy. In systematic desensitization it has been shown that muscle relaxation and the hierarchy of stimulus items are not the key curative factors. Jaffe (1968) showed how induced expectation of success (i.e. suggestion) was more powerful than the treatment itself. The placebo group with the expectation of success fared better than the treatment group without the expectation of success.

The invention of what later came to be called the standard frame for the practice of psychoanalysis evolved out of slowly trying different clinical methods over time. This contrasts sharply with the structured teaching for the general population that follows after the death of the founding teacher/intellect. Consequent generations are not exposed to the original teachings and in addition may not have the same motivation or capacities than those that were formed closely after the original invention.

So the standard treatment, like standardized testing in general education, is a way of transmitting and disseminating a theory and a practice (as well as information) to a wider population. Here an inverse relation can be observed between professional education and clinical practice. The standard treatment allows for structured training for a larger group of clinicians who may have a more technical and less intellectual focus in their cognitive orientation. At the same time, as already mentioned, a standard treatment also makes it more difficult to shape the theory and the practice to changing times, populations, and settings. In general education, we also have the example of Finland where they eliminated all standardized testing in education and saw a rise in educational outcomes for their student population. Rather than study the logic of the test, memorize or guess answers to multiple choice questions, students had to know and be able to explain the answers to questions.

There is an inherent conflict or contradiction between invention or innovation and tradition, the individual leader and the group, and between invention and practice according to the standard operating procedures outlined by manuals and handbooks. Furthermore institutionalized practices that come to be identified with the tradition may come to oppose the spirit of the original teachings or invention. On the other hand Winnicott was right when he said, "it is not possible to be original except on a basis of tradition."

Psychically or 'emotionally' organizations both claim to steadfastly obey established knowledge yet at the same time oppose and marginalize the inventive minds that created the knowledge in the first place. The power of organizations is that they get to have it both ways: both obey and defy the founders at the same time (an obsessive symptom, therefore).

In this sense, the non-standard frame is the source of the standard one rather than the other way around. In addition, creative individuals will always experiment and practice beyond the limits set by current standard practices because otherwise science and knowledge would not evolve.

Freud invented a standard treatment out of prior practices that did not conform to the new standards he developed, yet continued to use the new method in non-standard ways. Nonetheless, Freud did not have a framework to account for the contradictions between the standard and non-standard ways within his practice.

However, as argued by many in the philosophy of science, mainstream science always needs to tolerate rogue elements in their midst because new ideas could not evolve otherwise that could be consequently proven to be true within the framework of science.

The formalization of the non-standard frame was, essentially, Lacan's contribution to the practice and effectiveness of psychoanalysis. Lacan wrote "Variations on the Standard Treatment" back in 1953 (Lacan, 2006 [1966]). In this paper he stated: "A psychoanalysis, whether standard or not, is the treatment one expects from a psychoanalyst" (p. 274).

The standard treatment was further developed and institutionalized under the IPS and the leadership of Anna Freud to protect the legacy of Freud and in the process made the standard treatment the official statement regarding the practice of psychoanalysis. While establishing the standard-treatment the IPS intended to be "more Freudian than Freud" and treated Freud's unorthodox or non-standard methods as Freud's idiosyncrasies, lack of a personal analysis, and being the first analyst. By the same token, they crystallized and froze Freud's actual idiosyncrasies into the rigid structure of an international organization.

Institutions, as sociologists have pointed out, often gain a life of their own and have a self-preservation instinct, operating according to the prescriptions of their leaders, but in the process rigidifying and distorting the qualities that their leaders possess. Freud, was well aware of this fact and is reported to have said, "My pupils are more orthodox that I" [cited by Roazen, 1975, p. 401].

Although many analysts in every generation have practiced in non-standard ways and analysts in sessions do what fits and is necessary despite the official standard treatment, such non-standard methods remain uninvestigated, and rarely have been reported.

I realize that there are many historical nuances regarding the standard treatment that historians might dispute, but I believe that the distinction between standard and non-standard holds across time, and not only has heuristic value, but is also a very important axis or vertex from which to examine the question of psychoanalytic practice in both public and private settings.

Octave Mannoni in France gave a famous example regarding what he called the Procrustean couch: if someone does not fit into the frame then you cut an arm, then a leg, etc. This is how many analysts from IPA institutes are perceived outside psychoanalysis. Analysts are perceived as only wanting to help patients that are good candidates for psychoanalysis or work with diagnoses that fit into the psychoanalytic frame. Although this may be relevant for private practice with a less disturbed population, it severely handicaps psychoanalytic work within institutions and with minorities.

Although it is a good practice to be able to determine which treatments are good or effective for what conditions, it is also true that the mental health professions have the responsibility of helping all potential patients requesting services in institutions, not only those who are helped by traditional psychoanalysis or the standard treatment. Psychoanalysts are often perceived as only wanting to help the interesting, insightful, wealthy, and higher functioning patients who fit into the frame of traditional psychoanalysis.

As stated above, the non-standard treatment has always existed alongside the standard treatment. In addition, the distinction between standard and non-standard treatment differs from the distinction often made between psychoanalysis and psychotherapy. Although psychoanalytic psychotherapy is often perceived as having wider applicability than psychoanalysis, the former is still perceived as only appropriate for a less disturbed and higher-functioning population. In this sense, the notion of a non-standard treatment or a multiform criterion for the practice of psychoanalysis is directly related to the need to apply psychoanalysis to a wider range of clinical populations.

There are certain rules that any meaningful psychoanalysis should follow such as confidentiality, satisfaction of an inmost request for unconscious knowing, patient's ability and willingness to speak and free associate without holding back, and the analyst's ability to listen without judgments. Those are the factors that we can and should control. However at the same time we should not forget about the human factor of undetermination, unpredictability, and an element of surprise, that are also important parts of the treatment. We do not know in what words or language the unconscious of the analysand will be ciphered or what words analysands will use to constitute themselves as subjects of the unconscious. Some of these will be known but repressed/forgotten and some of them will be new inventions emerging from the Real unconscious of the subject.

In analysis every significant object in the subject's speech will stem from a past or unconscious relation between the subject and the other/Other. Although nothing new, the repressed unconscious manifests as a random and automatic production/formation of the unconscious and of speech. As Lacan suggests in Seminar XXIII, every object is defined by a relation between x and y, and the relation itself can be described by a z or an epithet which is a word or name expressing a characteristic. However, the *objet a* in or on the Real is solitary or a singularity, because it is empty of inherent nature, of concept and signifier (lack of a concept and a signifier). This latter object will require the invention of a *sinthome* or a process of nomination to be named and drained from the Real.

"All I have got is what I have not got", said once an analysand to Winnicott (2011 [1971], p. 124). She later added "'And what will you do about it?' As Winnicott remained silent, she said, 'Oh, I see.' Thereupon, Winnicott made a comment full of humanity and humility: 'I am silent because I don't know what to say.'" In relation to what the analysand said Winnicott disclosed his own lack rather than revealing what he had to give that the analysand was demanding. In several occasions Winnicott did not hide what he did not know and he thought it was important for the analyst not to remain in a position of omnipotence.

However, in this example there is a difference between lack in the analyst and the analysand. Winnicott accepts his lack or not 'having' anything to say, while the analysand demands that the analyst fill the lack as presented by the analysand. The analysand is conveying her fundamental fantasy that the Other is lacking. Now the lack in the analysand's case that Winnicott is discussing, refers to the environment mother. Apparently this analysand had sustained early losses that were traumatic beyond the normal loss associated with separation, the loss of the breast in weaning, of feces, or the not having the imaginary phallus that takes place in normal neurosis.

One could read this case as either the analysand wanting the analyst to repair or fill the hole left by the real (small r) absence of the object (privation), or as the analysand wanting the analyst to give her something that neither she nor the analyst's has and that the analyst can only promise to give under false pretenses. This is an inevitable and necessary absence or emptiness/lack (symbolic castration) that has to be accepted rather than filled or treated as a defect. Since the latter is an inevitable existential condition that no adequate environment will ever prevent, this is a form of suffering any subject will have to endure. The analysand accepts this when faced with Winnicott's lack of response.

The singular case is to be distinguished from a subject's sense of their particular uniqueness or false sense of autonomy from the group. The group here would refer to social norms, group identities, and statistical norms that can be given and revealed by group reports, surveys, structured interviews, questionnaires, and statistics. In psychoanalysis, the Other of the unconscious occupies the place of the group report, which to simplify things a little would stand for language and the law but also the cultural heritage, environment, religion, geography etc. that a particular person is born into.

The singular or a singularity refers not to an alleged unique trait of distinction such as the specialness of a proper name as distinguished from a common noun. A unique narcissistic object or trait of the subject, for example, would stem from unconscious desire or from the unconscious desires and objects that the subject represented for significant others in the subject's life. A singularity instead refers to a solitary *unary trace*, or an often non-sensical letter, word, holophrase, or name coming from the Real experience of a subject and that can be isolated from a symbolic signifying chain.

During the course of analysis the analysand is faced with a choice. In the case of the Wolf-man, Freud (1918) said that analysands can be cured only if they want to be cured. One can enter analysis like buying a train ticket for an unknown destination but buying the ticket does not oblige the potential traveller to actually travel aboard the train. The decision making process is independent from the Other. The Other provides the structure and context for a choice, and although the Other constitutes the subject, the subject is also self-constituted through particular choices, actions, and fantasies.

The Name of the Father is a fundamental signifier of the Symbolic order, in the same way that in set theory the empty set grounds the succession of whole numbers. However, the analysand needs to arrive at the key signifiers and experiences that organize their own singular signifying world. Eventually Lacan replaced his concept of the-Name-of the-Father (the one that separates the mother from the child and symbolizes their relationship) with the later idea of the function of the father which is nothing else but a nonsensical signifier, detached from the chain of signifiers, one that we invent ex nihilo in the process of analysis. Such signifier is a different Other or the NoF emerging from the Real.

Let me give you an example from the beginning of the middle phase of an analysis. An analysand reported two related dreams. In the first he is hiding in the dark corner of a shed from men that are searching for him while mocking him at the same time. In the second dream, he is under siege by an army of men. In his associations to the dreams, he made reference to the father figure in a tv show meant to convey an ideal father. In contrast he referred to himself as a weak version of that. He also noted that he had many dreams where he is being attacked or he is attacking other men often violently.

This analysand came from a family with a history of family violence such that in one instance the mother used a shot gun to put a bullet through the father's hand. The father was a drunk and a poor provider, and the analysand was a good boy and a son of the mother, who told him he should not be anything like the father. Yet the analysand turned out to have vocational and work-related problems, as well as two accidents that disabled him from being able to be a good provider for his family. He is often understated and non-aggressive, yet wished to be more aggressive specially towards other men by whom he felt overpowered.

The third association to the dream may be the charm. He reported being told at some point by his parents, that a neighbor sexually abused his sister. The neighbor would take him and his sister to his house after school, because his parents were still at work or busy. The sexual abuse of the sister happened in a shed behind the house. The analysand denied having survivor's guilt or feeling responsible for not preventing the sister's abuse from taking place. He said he was too young to know anything about it.

The symbolic work of analysis is to create links between random associations the analysand produces within the psychoanalytic session. In this case, he is linking weak father, with a weak man under attack, and most remotely with an identification with his sister being under assault in a shed. The word shed provides the link between the dream image, and what happened to the sister in a shed in his childhood. The layer that is most repressed is that being a 'weak' man in relationship to aggressive men is being equated to being a small girl under sexual attack by an older man, and that he is considering himself a girl like his sister. Weak girl is being equated to weak man or father.

In terms of technique, the analyst simply marks the borders of the unknown unconscious area and asks the analysand to associate by asking the question, for example, of what comes to his mind about the dream putting him in the position of his sister. If the analysand is not ready or balks at the content of the material, the analyst would be content with waiting until the analysand is ready or his unconscious produces more material to this effect. Finally, the symbolic work of analysis represents something of the psychical, beyond the necessary telling of a traumatic experience. The difficult telling or reporting of sexual abuse, for example, takes place on a different level of narration or of the signifying chain more acceptable to and consistent with social norms.

The theory would formulate that the analysand's unconscious is equating femininity with an imaginary form of 'weakness' (both males and females are feminine in this instance), and strong masculinity with an imaginary form of masculine strength or domination (in males or females). Both forms of weakness are victims of imaginary castration while strength and aggressiveness is linked to an unbarred and uncastrated form of masculinity. In the analysand's mind, there is no category for symbolically castrated masculinity or femininity. The men or the mother are either violently aggressive, or the sister, women, and men are weak victims to more powerful masculine predators whether male or female.

New names and words will have to be discovered or invented to symbolize something about a productive form of symbolic femininity, and a Real femininity beyond symbolic castration. The same can be said about men and the father. There will be no Real femininity for a man in the Symbolic register, but a man may access the Real in other ways that are also available to women (jouissance of meaning, or of the mystic, for example).

For a woman, and femininity in the Real and the Symbolic, the *sinthome* will be found in the ways that a woman makes do with the lack of a signifier for femininity. For example one analysand may have identified with a masculine signifier such as wearing men's boots. Since as a female she is not entirely comfortable wearing men's boots (a symptom of her rejection of femininity) because they put her at odds with her gender, she also has five bins full of women shoes, that point to some signifier of femininity that she also is not entirely comfortable with. The latter experimentation will become her *sinthome.*

The process of symbolization/nomination will invent something new at the site of the symptom in the analysand's psyche (a victim to other men) to repair the damage done by the failures of the paternal/parental metaphor (the father's irresponsibility and drunkness and the mother's aggressiveness). This could not take place without first addressing the symbolic, psychical aspect of this patient's makeup.

The multiform criterion for the practice of analysis represents an operational mode that aims to recognize and focus on the evanescent pulsation of the unconscious (opening and closing during sessions and different phases of analysis) within a different temporal dimension of speech. Different conditions (standard or non standard) may help or hinder the manifestation of the unconscious in analysis. The unconscious manifests in the here and now of a session and within the singularity of the frame for each treatment. On a case-by-case basis each treatment may have a variable length and frequency of sessions and treatment.

Sometimes the analyst will speak more and sometimes speak less, sometimes ask the right questions, or make necessary and contraposing citations of the analysand, and sometimes let the analysand speak freely without interruption. Sometimes the analyst may focus on conscious material if this is all the analysand may speak about, but this is a strategy within the transference to help bring out unconscious material. The analyst must meet the analysand where the analysand is at rather than always staying silent and waiting for the analysand to speak about something that they may never speak about or they may never know that they knew without the help of the analyst. More than having objectives or goals for each treatment, or having a manual or a frame to treat all individuals alike, analysts need a way to track the analysand's singular track or path leading to symptom reduction/resolution, to a know-how regarding the sympton, and to a capability for benevolent jouissance and unconscious knowing.

This is why standarization is problematic because it leads to the false conclusion that it contains the origin of the succession when in fact it may not. Lacan's use of the Real, and the scansion of speech and session was his way of re-establishing the Real of the unconscious within the Symbolic series rather than simply replacing the Real for a standard Symbolic.

The two systems of non-standard and standard analysis (S_1 and S_2) are represented in Table 10.1.

It is possible that the two sides of the table are equal despite the fact that they contain different elements. We are not saying by any means that the standard and non-standard forms of analyses are identical, but if they lead to the same result we could come to the conclusion that they are equal. Although some elements are shared and some are not, both systems are equal or the final logical result may be the same. However, obviously our bet, and that of the Lacan school, is that, more often than not, the non-standard will be more effective than the standard treatments that can lead to exceedingly long and protracted analysis, and to the downfall of psychoanalysis as a treatment method, therefore.

Table 10.1 The two systems of non-standard and standard analysis (S_1 and S_2)

Non-standard analysis	Standard analysis
Transference analysis and interventions within the transference	Transference interpretations
No fixed length of session	45–50 minute length of session
No fixed length of treatment	Fixed length of treatment
No fixed sitting arrangement	Exclusive use of the couch
Possible variation in the location of the treatment (i.e. use of phone, online video sessions, etc.)	Exclusive use of the private office
Scansion of speech	Free association
Going from the unknown to the unknown	Going from the unknown to the known
Personal psychoanalysis	

Lacanians bet on the idea that the scansion/punctuation of speech and session increases the effectiveness of the session, and prevents stalemates and idle repetitive speech in analysis. In contrast, the standard frame may lead to stalemates, impasses or interminable analyses. However, to be consistent the non-standard frame has to include a standard frame as a possible variation in the treatment. Otherwise, the non-standard frame paradoxically becomes a standard frame. Conversely, a standard frame that allows for the variations of a non-standard analysis, can no longer be said to be a standard analysis, although the latter could still be practiced depending on the singular analysand and the context.

There are those who argue that only technique or the frame is fundamental for psychoanalysis or clinical practice in general. This empirical perspective is often associated with a complete rejection of theory, or is at least linked to the argument that theory is secondary to practice or therapeutic relationships. On the other side, there are those who argue that theory is necessary to work with the singular case, since technique may be applicable to one case but not to another.

Another way to consider this binary is whether the psychoanalyst or psychoanalytic theory guides a general psychiatric or psychological doctor of the mind who has many tools in his/her 'bag of tricks', or if, on the other hand, a psychoanalyst is one among many mental health professionals using specific techniques derived from empirical studies supporting a variety of competing theories of mind and behavior.

I distinguish among three approaches to theory. The first can be closely linked to what Lacan called the 'cock and bull' story line, the ideology that stays close to ordinary narratives that are contextually specific or limited and that advances particular cognitive interests or defenses against psychoanalysis. This type of theory is not far removed from what the Frankfurt school called instrumental reason and can be described as idiosyncratic in nature.

The second type of theory, which could be called Symbolic, is one that uses language and logic and a battery of signifiers to describe a structure operative within human experience. Reason here can be formal, critical, or dialectical but in general is linked to the history of ideas as well as to science and to other disciplines of knowledge. Finally, there is the theory that captures the thing itself in the Real and describes the jouissance of both the subject and the Other using nonsensical sounds, numbers, or invented words.

We argue that psychoanalysis has to make use of all of these three levels of reason and that psychoanalytic theories can be classified according to the extent that they use and are embedded within and across these levels of rationality. Freud and the first generation of disciples, as well as ego psychology and object relations, used the first two levels of rationality, while Bion and Lacan, especially, used all three.

With regards to the relationship between theory and technique at least two positions or perspectives are possible. There are those who argue that all new evidence-based techniques are extensions and repackaging of psychoanalytic ideas and techniques able to be sold in the market place under a new brand.

On the other hand, there are those who argue that specific techniques should be used and labeled following the empirical studies that they are derived from, and that these techniques though they may appear to be similar to traditional psychoanalytic ideas, are entirely different and the two should not be confused. CBT, DBT, motivational interviewing, harm reduction, and mentalization, are some of the examples that immediately come to mind. We do not agree with this position, for the reasons discussed above regarding the logic of singularity and the two types of reason needed for psychoanalytic observations.

Table 10.2 shows how many of the 'modern' techniques are derived from psychoanalytic ideas.

To summarize I would like to use the basic schema of Lacan's graph of desire to represent the different categories used in this chapter. I am only using three of the overall lines included in the graph. In addition, the mathemes at the edges (both inside and outside the circles) are ignored as not being that relevant for the current purposes. For a more detailed exposition of the graph of desire please refer to Romanowicz and Moncayo (2015).

Lacanian psychoanalysis encompasses the three vectors used: one vertical and two horizontal (Fig. 10.1).

The vertical vector (of desire) begins with the clinical problem presentation and the patient or analysand's speech and ends in the outcome expected from applied psychoanalysis. The symbols that Lacan uses for the vertical vector are the divided subject or $ (clinical problem) and the ego ideal or I[A] (the ideal aims or outcomes of treatment). Pure psychoanalysis represents the upper floor horizontal vector going from left to right and associated with free association and interventions on the unconscious signifying chain (from the signifier of lack in the unconscious to the demands of the drive and the questions of desire).

The lower level represents the manifest narratives and problems/statements addressed by the psychotherapist and most commonly associated with psychotherapy. In the example used above, the symbolization of the sister's trauma and story would represent the lower level signifying chain, while the signifying chain linking the shed with issues of

Table 10.2 Many of the 'modern' techniques are derived from psychoanalytic ideas

Psychoanalysis	Group reports
Sadistic super ego is in conflict with reality ego	That you will never feel better or that you are always depressed is not a realistic idea (CBT)
Suspension of judgment	Radical acceptance (DBT)
Do not give advice	Do not tell patients to stop using substances and instead motivate them to want to stop using substances (Motivational interviewing)

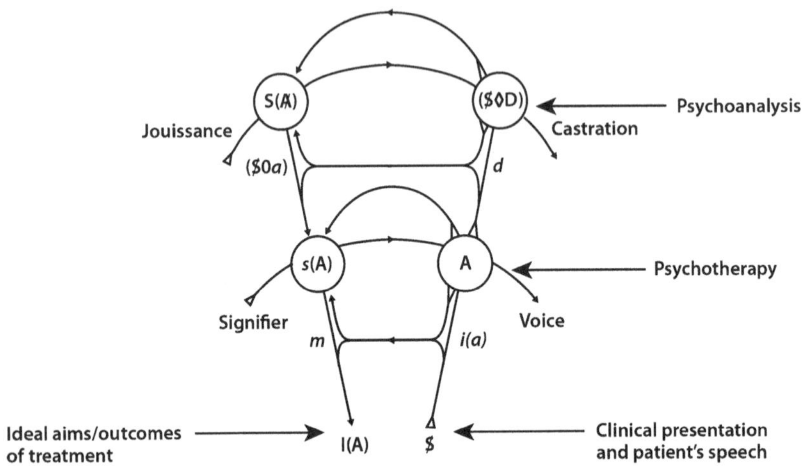

Fig. 10.1 Complete graph of desire. Romanowicz and Moncayo (2015)

'sexuation' or conflicting gender identifications and the question of a weak or strong father, and aggressiveness in relationships, are part of the upper level of the signifying chain.

The standard treatment and the non-standard treatment for the practice of psychoanalysis may take place in either of the two levels and may or may not achieve the aims of applied psychoanalysis. Finally, non-psychoanalytic psychotherapy would entirely exclude and bypass the upper floor of the graph. Although both psychoanalysis and psychotherapy may reach the end point of the vertical vector, psychoanalysis leads to self-knowledge and to unknown knowing or unconscious knowing, an expanded awareness or psychic state, and conscious knowledge of the unconscious. Finally, pure psychoanalysis (in standard or non-standard formats) may lead to more long-lasting results and lower relapse rates but through what Lacan calls the identification with the *sinthome*.

What Lacan calls identification with the *sinthome* at the end of analysis for our purposes may be simply defined as a modification of the psychical/characterological structure of the subject as a result of the work with the symptom in treatment. The change in characterological structure leads to the subject taking responsibility for the symptom which in the process become *sinthomes* rather than simple symptoms. The *sinthome* becomes a source of unconscious knowing. There is a different qualitative relationship to the symptom instead of the symptom being quantitatively eradicated. Difficult characterological traits may still be there, but are now ego-dystonic and a source of ongoing jouissance and transformation for the subject.

According to Lacan the post treatment effects of analysis refer not to the identification with the analyst as a good object, as termination is understood within object relations theory. The analysand may identify and want to be like the analyst as an ego ideal, but this form of identity will be a form of compliance with the treatment as opposed to representing a form of 'unbeing' in the Real subject. The nomination process and jouissance associated with the *sinthome* will support the function of the *sinthome* as a source of unconscious knowledge. This is more fundamental than internalizing the ego of the analyst as a good object.

This work with the *sinthome* continues after analysis and would explain the post-termination lower relapse rates. Knowing how to work with the *sinthome*, or caring for the *sinthome* in the service of personal development, is a very different thing than thinking that you are cured or enlightened once and for all. The latter in fact is a fantasy caused by our gaining ideas, ideas of self-improvement, and in general the instrumental and humanistic culture of contemporary society.

Conclusion

In this chapter I have examined the relations between the non-standard and standard treatment or applied and pure forms of psychoanalysis. Applied psychoanalysis, the multiform criterion, or the non-standard treatment, can be differentiated from the standard treatment as well as from psychoanalytic psychotherapy. I believe that only with a well-grounded theory and craft, psychoanalysis can be effectively practiced both in standard and non-standard ways.

References

Badiou, A., & Roudinesco, E. (2014). *Jacques Lacan, Past and Present: A Dialogue*. New York: Columbia University Press.

Busch, F. N., Milrod, B. L., & Sandberg, L. S. (2013). A Study Demonstrating Efficacy of a Psychoanalytic Psychotherapy for Panic Disorder: Implications for Psychoanalytic Research, Theory, and Practice. *Journal of the American Psychoanalytic Association, 57*(1), 131–148. 2009 Feb.

Freud, S. (1918 [1914]). *From the History of an Infantile Neurosis*. SE, 17, 1–123. London: Hogarth Press.

Hicks, R. D. (1907). *Aristotle De Anima with Translation, Introduction, and Notes*. London: Cambridge University Press.

Jaffe, L. W. (1968). *Non-specific Treatment Factors and Deconditioning in Fear Reduction* (Unpublished doctoral dissertation). University of Southern California.

Lacan, J. (2006 [1966]). *Ecrits* (B. Fink, Trans.). New York: W.W. Norton.

Leichsenring, F., & Rabung, S. (2008). Effectiveness of Long-Term Psychodynamic Psychotherapy: A Meta-analysis. *Journal of the American Medical Association, 300*, 1551–1565.

Leichsenring, F., & Rabung, S. (2009). Analyzing Effectiveness of Long-Term Psychodynamic Psychotherapy Reply. *Journal of the American Medical Association, 301*, 932–933.

Levy, R. A., Ablon, J. S., & Kächele, H. (2011). *Psychodynamic Psychotherapy Research: Evidence-Based Practice and Practice-Based Evidence*. New York: Springer.

Miller, J. A. (2015). *Pure Psychoanalysis, Applied Psychoanalysis, and Psychotherapy*. http://www.lacan.com/lacinkXX2.htm. Last accessed Feb 2015.

Moncayo, R. (2017). *Lalangue, Sinthome, Jouissance, and Nomination. A Reading Companion and Commentary on Lacan's Seminar XXIII*. London: Karnac Books Ltd.

Moncayo, R., & Romanowicz, M. (2015). *The Real Jouissance of Uncountable Numbers. The Philosophy of Science Within Lacanian Psychoanalysis*. London: Karnac.

O'Conner, P. (1999). *Words Fail Me*. New York: Houghton Harcourt Publishing.

Pennebaker, J. (1995). *Emotion, Disclosure, and Health*. Washington, DC: American Psychological Association.

Pennebaker, J. (1997). *Opening Up: The Healing Power of Confiding in Others*. New York: Guilford.

Roazen, P. (1975). *Freud and His Followers*. New York: Knopf.

Romanowicz, M., & Moncayo, R. (2015). Going Beyond Castration in the Graph of Desire. *The Letter (The Irish Journal for Lacanian Psychoanalysis), 58*(Spring), 31–58.

Schedler, J. (2010). The Efficacy of Psychodynamic Psychotherapy. *American Psychologist, 65*(2), 98–109.

Steiner, H. (1977). Freud Against Himself. *Perspectives in Biology and Medicine, 20*(4), 510–527.

Winnicott, D. (2011 [1971]). Transitional Objects and Transitional Phenomena. In *Reading Winnicott*. London: Routledge.

11

The Lacanian School as an Organizational Structure

Introduction

Thirty-seven years after his death, the work of Jacques Lacan remains clinically disputed yet theoretically vindicated. The practice of Lacanian analysis is still disputed within IPA institutes who are struggling to reconcile the growing popularity of Lacan and Lacanian analysis with the initial decision that excluded him from the organization. Morever, Lacanian clinical practice may be disputed within IPA psychoanalysis, but this fact is small in comparison to how psychoanalysis at large is clinically disputed within evidence-based practices.

As mentioned in the previous chapter, at some point,

> The word psychoanalysis or Freud or Freudian psychoanalysis became a taboo word within the clinic of evidence-based practices. There are many reasons for this being the case despite the fact that nowadays brief psychodynamic psychotherapy has joined the ranks of evidence-based-practices in mental or so-called "behavioral" health.

This chapter has been co-authored by Dany Nobus and sections of it first appeared in Nobus' (2016) paper on Lacan and organizational theory.

R. Moncayo, *Knowing, Not-Knowing, and Jouissance*, The Palgrave Lacan Series,
https://doi.org/10.1007/978-3-319-94003-8_11

Although there is empirical evidence that psychoanalysis is effective as a treatment (as argued in the previous chapter), Lacanian psychoanalysis is less disputed within the general culture because it is a new form of psychoanalysis, and science must remain open to new treatments that have not been quantitatively tested.

Lacanian psychoanalysis follows from a different form of rationality and epistemology as already argued. The experience and clinical effect of psychoanalysis is a singularity that can only be verified on a case by case basis and then with difficulty due to the social, ethical, and legal problems involved in disclosing information associated to case histories. The material disclosed in analytical sessions is not limited to social narratives and histories of abuse that could be disclosed to the public and are even disclosed to the public in TV talk shows.

The decline of psychoanalysis is also due to internal reasons, one of which affects Lacanian psychoanalysis and the other does not. The first follows from a dogmatic theoretical position by which we mean not the enumeration of first principles, which is inevitable in science, nor the provision of proofs, but the refusal to consider other schools of thought within or outside psychoanalysis.

The second internal reason for the decline of psychoanalysis affects psychoanalysis but not Lacanian psychoanalysis. Mainstream psychoanalysis remains dogmatic with respect to the frame for treatment which was the main reason for expelling Lacan from the IPA. In this Lacanian psychoanalysis is revolutionary and may coincide with the external critiques of psychoanalysis. The scansion and citation of speech in analysis, and the scansion of the length of the session represent a renewed practice of interpretation that goes a long way in addressing the questioned effectiveness of psychoanalytic interpretations and insight as predictable conscious explanations of the unconscious that are not clinically efficient.

Although Lacan wanted his form of psychoanalysis to take root in North American soil, not only the difficulty of his texts, but also a dogmatic and colonialist attitude on the part of French and European psychoanalysts was not helpful in this regard. What helped establish the first Lacanian School of psychoanalysis in the US (LSP) twenty-six years ago, was the attempt not only to teach Lacanian psychoanalysis as a clinical practice, but also to apply Lacanian theory and practice to clinical work in institutions, to use and teach Lacanian theory in local universities, to dialogue with other forms of psychoanalysis, and to accept the local licensing laws for the various professions under which psychoanalysis can take place. At the same time, we are aware that the regulation of the profession can also have an adverse effect on its practice, since the restrictions of the Law do not encourage or support the rule of free association about topics, themes, and fantasies regulated and repressed by the Law. The state regulation of the profession has the effect of generating or enforcing a climate of conformity that may be inimical to the spirit of psychoanalysis.

Nowadays LSP is a functioning Lacanian school in the United States based in California and supporting the practice of Lacanian analysis across the country. Bruce Fink's translations of Lacan's work and Fink's own introductory texts have helped disseminate Lacanian analysis in the United States. Most Lacanian analysts in the US and UK are also licensed and professionally trained clinicians. In the UK, CFAR (Centre for Freudian Analysis and Research) forms clinicians who are then authorized to practice once they finish the requirements for training within the institution. This is a better system than the licensing laws of the US, that require a host of professional bureaucrats, and an industry of experts that live off the regulation of the practicing professional clinician. Given the trajectory of psychoanalysis as a child of Europe, psychoanalysts in Europe were in a better position to mount legal challenges to the attempts by the State to regulate the profession.

In this chapter, we would like to look at the Lacanian school as an organization, beginning with a review of Lacan's trajectory in attempting to develop a new psychoanalytic organization.

Lacan's theories have gone from strength to strength in academic departments of literature, cultural studies, modern languages, linguistics and rhetoric, media and communication studies, women's and gender studies, philosophy and film theory. The versatile applicability of his concepts as solid tools for critical analysis is also demonstrated in the widest range of disciplines outside the traditional human and social sciences, and seems to gain more and more momentum daily, with architects, legal scholars, criminologists, educational scientists, theologians and classicists now also engaging with his work (see e.g. Beattie, 2013; Caudill, 1997; Cho, 2009; Hendrix, 2006; Jagodzinski, 2005; Miller, 2007; Milovanovic, 2003).

Since the late 1990s, Lacan's notions have also started to gain momentum in organization research, critical management theory, business studies and public administration scholarship, on both sides of the Atlantic. Many of the new Lacanians in these fields have demonstrated how key Lacanian concepts such as the mirror stage, the divided subject, the *objet a*, desire, *jouissance*, fantasy, and discourse can be used productively in order to understand, inter alia, how organizations function and become dysfunctional (e.g. Arnaud, 2002), how individuals operating within organizations maintain their professional identities and develop certain types of working relationships with their colleagues (e.g. Arnaud & Vanheule, 2007; Driver, 2009b, 2009c; Harding, 2007; Kosmala & Herrbach, 2006), how authentic leadership is established (e.g. Costas & Taheri, 2012), how work-related problems such as envy, stress and burnout may be addressed (e.g. Bicknell & Liefooghe, 2010; Driver, 2014; Vanheule, Lievrouw, & Verhaeghe, 2003; Vanheule & Verhaeghe, 2004; Vidaillet, 2007), how strategic and operational change management may be facilitated (e.g. Driver, 2009a; Kenny, 2009), how practices of human resource management affect individuals at work (e.g. Johnsen & Gudmand-Høyer, 2010), how executive coaching and consulting can be tailored to subjective as well as collective needs (e.g. Arnaud, 2003), how entrepreneurship discourse is predicated upon the assumption of certain "work identities" (e.g. Jones & Spicer, 2005), how staff representatives react to the threat of factory closure (Vidaillet & Gamot, 2015), and how organizational processes are conditioned by broader socio-political and economic configurations (e.g. Bloom & Cederström, 2009; Fotaki, 2009; Glynos, 2011; Stavrakakis, 2008). If Lacan has not fully arrived yet in organization and critical management studies, then he is making serious headway as a theoretical force to be reckoned with.

If we restrict "organizational culture", then, to the classic structure of the corporate enterprise operating under economic conditions of high capitalism, Lacan indeed emerges as the anti-organizational psychoanalytic theorist par excellence. As an anti-humanist and a fierce critic of the adaptation paradigm in ego-psychology and related psychoanalytic models, Lacan was profoundly weary of any developmental, corrective and accumulative perspective on mental health, and of any clinical and theoretical outlook that regards the restoration of a patient's psychic economy and its return to a well-integrated state of stable equilibrium as a realistic aspiration (see e.g. Lacan, 1988 [1953–1954], p. 25; Lacan, 2006 [1953], p. 204; Van Haute, 2002). By extension, Lacan was extremely sceptical of any social system that inscribes progress and growth as the most advanced accomplishments into its discourse, because he did not believe that the outcomes (goods and services) of a production cycle can be fully achieved through regulatory frameworks (Lacan, 2006 [1968–1969], pp. 15–19).

Obviously, these points would apply to both theory and practice. The ideology of health and well-being is a humanistic approach that is deeply entrenched in the delivery of public mental health services within the United States. Fromm's humanistic psychoanalysis and the humanistic theories of Abraham Maslow and Carl Rogers have been influential in this regard. Lacan would be critical of these developments as having lost the creative edge of the Freudian analysis of the Unconscious.

Ego psychology within psychoanalysis advocates the ego's adaptive, integrative, and synthetic functions that promote a notion of psychical equilibrium within the context of social reality and the reality principle. This approach blends well with psychiatry as a social institution that promotes biological health and normal or normative social behaviour.

What is lost in these approaches is a critical perspective on normal behaviour, and an idealistic/humanistic philosophy serves as a defence against the importance of psychopathology and the symptom for personal development. Lacanian psychoanalysis is centred on the Real of the Unconscious rather than on a humanistic ideal or a historically determined social reality.

However, Lacanians have not abandoned Freud's insistence on the transformations of the symptom and psychoanalysis as a treatment for psychical suffering (applied psychoanalysis). The observations of psychoanalysis, although empirical and clinical, are singular and apply to each subject in which psychoanalysis is reinvented as a practice and a theory. Clinical outcomes can be measured according to symptom index scales in the areas of work and relationships. However, Lacan did abandon measuring psychoanalytic outcomes based on the ability to maintain relationships as is commonly the case within mainstream psychoanalysis and psychiatry (DSM's social and occupational objectives). If anything, social outcomes of treatment nowadays have to take into account the realities of relationships in contemporary society where many marriages end in failure and where Freud's developmental ideal of joining love and the sexual drive no longer holds.

What replaces the notion of a normative relationship is the realization that the human problem of an ideal rapport between the sexes does not exist. People may choose to make do or not with whatever relationships in which the *sinthome* may be implicated. In addition, the other side of the failure of the rapport between man and woman (male or female), is the proposition that "*Il y a d'Lun*" (the One 'ex-sists'). A singular subject may find equilibrium not in a relationship but in being "All-alone". This is not a narcissistic isolated individual but rather a singular subject linked to others through symbolic links and the Real that forges them. If Lacan has a developmental ideal it is through the subject of the Real of his later work that makes accord or creates new links and a new Borromean structure.

In line with this, Lacan did consider how the "anti-organizational" forms of lack, loss, and waste could be built into the walls of an alternative organization, how organizational life could be re-built, as it were, upon the foundations of incompleteness, as a non-totalizing entity in which hierarchical authority is balanced against a communal, libertarian and solidarity culture of exchange.

Esprit de Corps

In the late Summer of 1945, Lacan spent five weeks in England, during which period he visited Hatfield House in Hertfordshire, which at the time was a specialized centre for the rehabilitation of former prisoners-of-war and veterans. Still a psychiatrist, yet also already a psychoanalyst, what Lacan saw at Hatfield made a huge impression on him, so much so that upon his return to Paris he showered heaps of praise on this quintessentially English version of "democratic psychiatry": "To evaluate the importance of this work", Lacan declared to an audience of both French and British psychiatrists at the professional group of *L'évolution psychiatrique*, suffice it to say that 80% of the men […] choose freely to go through this gradual reintegration process [*éclusage*], where their stay is on average six weeks, but which can be shortened or prolonged upon their demand […]. "Psychiatry served to forge the instrument thanks to which Britain won the war; conversely, the war has transformed psychiatry in Britain" (Lacan, 2000 [1947], pp. 26–27).

Even more instructive than his visit to Hatfield was Lacan's long conversation with Wilfred R. Bion and John Rickman—"two men", he said, "of whom it can be said that the flame of creation burns in them" (ibid.: 15). During the Winter of 1942–'43, Bion had been put in charge of the rehabilitation of demoralized soldiers in the so-called "Training Wing" of the Northfield Military Hospital, near Birmingham (Harrison, 2000, p. 186).

Rather than reinforcing the Wing's iron army discipline, and actively preparing the soldiers for their swift return to military service, which had often seemed to result in an exacerbation of their neurotic symptoms, Bion helped the men re-focus their energies on the accomplishment of specific group tasks and the management of inter-personal relationships. Rather than treating the soldiers' neurotic conditions as individual illnesses, Bion decided to turn neurosis itself into the collective enemy, thus re-creating a positive *esprit de corps* characterised by shared loyalty, solidarity, fellowship, and an implicit sense of duty amongst the patients who became willing to accept responsibilities.

Lacan thought this so-called "first Northfield experiment" to be absolutely brilliant. Speaking to *L'évolution psychiatrique*, he stated: "[T]he lively details of this experience […] seem to me to be pregnant with a birth of sorts that is a new outlook opening upon the world" (Lacan, 2000 [1947], p. 19). But he did not stop there. Apart from complimenting the way in which English psychiatrists had succeeded in tackling the problem of war neurosis in new and imaginative ways, Lacan also applauded Bion's so-called "leaderless group project", which had been conducted some years before the first Northfield experiment, under the auspices of the War Office Selection Boards. As Bion put it, during the experiment "it was the duty of the observing officers to watch how any given man was reconciling his personal ambitions, hopes and fears with the requirements exacted by the group for its success" (Bion, 1946, p. 78).

Neither the observing officers, nor the advising psychiatrists, nor Bion himself for that matter, were acting upon a position of authoritarian leadership, but rather "suspended" their leadership in favour of releasing the group's own internal dynamics, thus also questioning its propensity to expect shotgun solutions to be delivered by identified leaders. Reflecting upon the experiments and justifying the idea of "suspended leadership", Bion later commented: "The group always make it clear that they expect me to act with authority as the leader of the group, and this responsibility I accept, though not in the way the group expect" (Bion, 1961 [1948–1951], p. 82). In his subsequent work with groups, Bion would consistently refuse to adopt a directive stance, instead allowing the group to evolve spontaneously and to follow its own internal laws, and only intervening when he believed he knew what was about to happen, which often left people in the group feeling puzzled and bemused.

Lacan strongly commended how English psychiatrists had made a major contribution to the war effort, but he was even more appreciative of the "democratic" principles supporting Bion's innovative recruitment device.

Firstly, rather than someone in an established position of authority recruiting and selecting the new officers, candidates are being given the opportunity to demonstrate in vivo what they are worth, and therefore to somehow self-select, in a situation of strict "fair play". Secondly, although the officers and psychiatrists assess individual contributions to the group task, they themselves only testify about what they have observed to a selection panel, so that theirs is only one voice among many, and the final decision is to a large extent based on what is conveyed in a "witness statement".

Thirdly, the objectivity and validity of the entire process are not driven by the controlled administration of psychometric tests or the use of conventional quantitative measures of physical and mental capacity, but rather by the careful elicitation and rigorous evaluation of strictly subjective phenomena (Lacan, 2000 [1947], pp. 22–24). It is these very principles that Lacan would endeavour to situate at the heart of the psychoanalytic training programme in the *École freudienne de Paris* (EFP), the organization which he himself founded in June 1964, some eight months after his exclusion from the International Psycho-Analytic Association (IPA).

Work Transference

Neither in his written texts, nor in any of his seminars did Lacan explicitly refer to Bion's work again, yet his most important contribution to organizational theory, namely his own foundation of the EFP and the fundamental pillars upon which it was built, was clearly inspired by Bion's experiments with leaderless groups and at Northfield. It should be mentioned, in this context, that up until the point when the EFP was established, Lacan had had a fair share of trouble with psychoanalytic institutions, not in the least with the IPA, from which he was definitively barred as a training analyst in November 1963 (Miller, 1977; Turquet, 2014).

The key events are worth recapitulating, here, if only because they once again illustrate that, contrary to what some scholars have claimed, Lacan had a lifelong interest in organizations, clearly positioned himself vis-à-vis a certain type of organizational culture, and typically argued in favour of an organizational structure that is commensurate with the nature of the task to be accomplished.

In 1934, whilst still in analytic training, Lacan joined the *Société Psychanalytique de Paris* (SPP), then the only psychoanalytic organization in France, and rapidly made his way through its ranks, becoming a full member in 1938 (Roudinesco, 1997 [1993], pp. 80, 86). When, after the second World War, the SPP resumed its activities, Lacan became a member of the SPP's "Teaching Committee" and in this capacity, he produced a paper outlining the procedures for the selection of new trainees, as well as the indicative contents of a psychoanalytic training programme, and the mechanisms for recognizing new psychoanalysts (Lacan, 1976 [1949]). The document was mainstream apart from the fact that Lacan did not de facto wish to exclude non-medically trained candidates from the psychoanalytic profession, and that he also proposed a certain de-centralization of power, allowing more members to participate in decision-making processes pertaining to candidate-selection and the delivery of teaching.

Then, during the Winter of 1952–'53, an acrimonious conflict erupted between Lacan and Sacha Nacht, the president of the SPP, around the organizational structure of a proposed psychoanalytic Training Institute, whereby Lacan's main reservations concerned the seemingly unassailable power of the Institute's directorate and the autocratic "examination" of the candidates' training by a sovereign group of self-appointed "officials". In the end, Lacan lost out and was forced to resign from the SPP, by which he also forfeited his membership of the IPA (Miller, 1976, p. 90). The minutes of the IPA business meeting of July 1953 indicate that Lacan's vehement attack on the Institute's hierarchical functioning may not have been the only problem, and that Lacan was also perceived as someone who would take unacceptable liberties with firmly established clinical rules. As Marie Bonaparte, by far the most prominent member of the SPP, put it to the IPA committee: "[O]ne of these members [Lacan] [...] promised to change his technique [of variable-length clinical sessions], but did not keep his promise" (Eissler, 1954, p. 272).

After the first split in the French psychoanalytic community, Lacan spent ten years delivering his weekly seminar at Sainte-Anne Hospital, as part of the analytic training programme of the newly created *Société Française de Psychanalyse* (SFP), whilst practicing as a psychoanalyst, entertaining people at his Summer house in Guitrancourt, and generally having fun. At the SFP, he did not occupy any important administrative or managerial positions, yet generally supported the new organization's request to be considered for re-admission to the IPA (Etchegoyen & Miller, 1996, p. 48).

However, throughout this period, Lacan also fired on all cylinders when considering the psychoanalytic establishment's practices and procedures, whereby he did not let an opportunity go by to ridicule the institutional hierarchy and its rigid, dogmatic attitudes towards analytic practice and training standards. Already in the 1953 "Rome Discourse", he suggested that the SPP's Training Institute was erected based on a "disappointing formalism that discourages initiative by penalizing risk and turns the reign of the opinion of the learned into a principle of docile prudence in which the authenticity of research is blunted even before it finally dries up" (Lacan, 2006 [1953], p. 199). With undisguised sarcasm, he went on to compare the Institute's conception of analytic training to 'that of a driving school which, not content to claim the privilege of issuing drivers' licenses, also imagines that it is in a position to supervise car construction' (ibid.: 200).

Lacan's finest moment came in 1956, in a paper published on the centenary of Freud's birth. Dissecting the so-called "situation" of psychoanalysis and the contemporary condition of psychoanalytic training programmes, he painted a hilarious satirical picture of the spurious distribution of power in the psychoanalytic establishment, in the great tradition of Swift and Rabelais. In "The Situation of Psychoanalysis and the Training of Psychoanalysts in 1956" (Lacan, 2006 [1956]), which remains one of Lacan's least studied papers, but also one of his most vehement repudiations of the hierarchical structure of (psychoanalytic) organizations, he designated those people who are in analysis as Little Shoes.

Little Shoes comply with institutional and clinical rules, do not dare to speak up for themselves outside the sessions, and generally follow the path imposed by the *soi-disant* or 'Sufficiencies', those who have successfully finished their analytic training and have been given full access to the psychoanalytic profession—psychoanalysts, as the Institution would call them. Lacan asserted that the Sufficiencies do not say much either, because self-sufficient as they are they do not feel the need to start a conversation or engage in discussion.

But then there are also the 'Beatitudes', in whom we can easily recognize the so-called "training analysts", and who have been appointed by the Sufficiencies, and put in charge (as superior members of the organization) of the Truly Necessary, i.e. those Little Shoes who do not come to see a psychoanalyst because they want to be relieved of some pressing personal problem but because they want to train as psychoanalysts.

In carefully laying out the stakes of his elaborate exposition, Lacan conceded that no psychoanalytic society can exist without Sufficiencies (practicing psychoanalysts), with the caveat that as a professional rank this position can only ever be reached asymptotically and therefore never be fully attained, so that Sufficiency is but the momentary occupation of a certain clinical position and not the definitive realisation of a certain professional stature. Put differently, for Lacan, analytic training is never fully finished, and no one should ever have the right or the duty to say that he or she *is* or has effectively become a psychoanalyst.

Critical as the presence of Sufficiencies may be for the survival of psychoanalytic organizations, Lacan was particularly disapproving, here, of the sovereign power they seem to have, not only in selecting the Truly Necessary (analytic trainees) and distinguishing them from the Little Shoes, but also in appointing the Beatitudes (training analysts) from their own kind, and deciding which of the Truly Necessary can become Sufficient on the basis of what the Beatitudes have managed to achieve with them. In short, Lacan disputed the doctrinal authority with which the psychoanalysts in the organization would concentrate all power within their own ranks, and exposed the psychoanalytic establishment as a ritualized, ceremonious and formulaic institution, not dissimilar to the self-perpetuating leadership of the Catholic priesthood or religious organizations.

Less than two months after Lacan was expelled from IPA and SPP he started again with a new seminar, in a new location and with a new audience. The topic was "the foundations of psychoanalysis", later to be modified into "the four fundamental concepts of psychoanalysis". At the beginning of the first lecture he could not resist reopening a barely healed wound, and so he started with the question "*En quoi y suis-je autorisé?*"—"What gives me the authority to do this?" or, as the English translator of the seminar renders the phrase: "Am I qualified to do so?" (Lacan, 1994 [1964], p. 1). Clearly, the problematic "authorization" in question did not simply concern Lacan's position as a lecturer but referred more specifically to his teaching about the foundations of psychoanalysis.

The question should thus be understood as: "What authorizes a psychoanalyst who has just been officially removed from his training position in a psychoanalytic organization to lecture on the basic principles of his discipline?" If the question was not entirely rhetorical, Lacan nonetheless decided that the "problem [be] deferred" (ibid.: 1). But not for too long. At the Summer solstice of 1964, Lacan created his own School, the *École Française de Psychanalyse* (EFP), subsequently to be renamed as the *École freudienne de Paris*. In the opening paragraphs of its "Founding Act" he emphasized that the organization (*l'organisme*) had been established to accomplish a programme of work (*un travail*), with three distinct aims: (1) restoring the cutting-edge truth of Freud's discovery; (2) returning the practice of psychoanalysis to its proper duty (*devoir*); and (3) denouncing the deviations and compromises that blunt and degrade psychoanalysis (Lacan, 1990 [1964], p. 97). Although he did not refer to Bion's distinction from the early 1950s between a productive work group and three inert basic-assumption groups (Bion, 1961 [1952]), Lacan thus set out with the explicit goal of forming a "work group", whose working objective or primary task (*objectif de travail*) consisted in a "movement of reconquest" (*mouvement de reconquête*) (Lacan, 1990 [1964], p. 97).

To ensure that the group would remain focused on the designated task and would not (as Bion would have had it) resort back to one or more "basic assumptions" (fight or flight; pairing or tactical political alliances against this or that; or idealization of a leader), Lacan proposed that the work be carried out by small groups of minimum three and maximum five people, *and* an additional person—the so-called "plus one"—who oversees selecting the concrete work topic, facilitating the discussion and determining the outcome of each individual group member's work (ibid.: 97). After some time, the small groups would be expected to permute, insofar as the individual members would be encouraged to leave to join another group. Lacan decided to call the small group a "cartel"—a name he glossed etymologically as being derived from the Latin *cardo*, meaning "hinge" (Lacan, 1990 [1964], p. 101; 1976 [1975], p. 221). It is important to note, here, that the cartel constitutes a temporary collective effort around the accomplishment of a set of specific individual tasks, from which the entire organization may benefit.

Being a member of a cartel (the essential work group) was also a necessary and sufficient condition for being a member of the School (Lacan, 1990 [1964], p. 100). In addition, Lacan stipulated that whoever is put in charge of "directing", be it the work of the cartels or (at a higher level) the work of the entire School, would not be occupying a chiefdom (*chefferie*), because of which he or she would then be given access to a higher rank. *Mutatis mutandis*, nobody in the School, regardless of rank and status, would be perceived as having been demoted if she or he engages in "base-level work" (ibid.: 97–98). Every individual enterprise (*enterprise personnelle*), regardless as to which position the individual occupies within the School, would moreover be subjected to institutional criticism and control, so that no hierarchical stratification makes someone inferior or superior, and a "circular organization" (*organisation circulaire*) is created (ibid.: 98).

The idea of the cartel was exceedingly simple and is redolent of the leaderless groups Bion set up when having to select new Army officers at the start of the second World War, with the proviso that in Lacan's School the cartels were not designed to select or recruit individuals, nor to facilitate any kind of therapeutic results, but to contribute to the accomplishment of the School's primary task. As such, the Lacanian cartel drew both on the leaderless group and Bion's "work group", whereby institutional leaders are placed in positions of "suspended" authority.

Although the concept and structure of the cartel was discussed extensively in the EFP, it did not prove nearly as controversial as Lacan's proposals for safeguarding the quality of the work and guaranteeing its transmission. If the cartel is the format and the mechanism by which the work is executed, then a certain regulatory framework is required to ensure that the work is captured, evaluated and communicated, internally as well as externally. What is required here, Lacan stated, is a "work transference" (*un transfert de travail*), which requires putting in place a system that enables the work to be transferred from one person to another, from one group to another, from the groups to the School, and from the School to its external environment (ibid.: 103). The notion of *transfert de travail* may very well be a hapax in Lacan's work, but should clearly be understood in connection with what, in his 1958 text on the direction of the treatment, he had already defined as *travail du transfert* (the work of transference) and *travail de transfert* (transference work), both terms adduced as translations of Freud's concept of *Durcharbeitung* (working through), which is meant to capture the most advanced part of the clinical psychoanalytic process (Freud, 1914, p. 155; Lacan, 2006 [1958], pp. 498, 526).

The two notions of the work of transference and transference work are two different notions that can be mistaken for one another. The same applies to the notion of transference love and love's transference in Freud. Transference is present in all relationships but has a technical meaning in the therapeutic relationship between analyst and analysand. The same is true of work transference and transference work. The first refers to the transference of work and of goods from one person to another in the work of the organization.

Transference proper is the transference of the Unconscious of the analysand (mainly sexual and aggressive fantasies, traumas, etc.) unto the analyst who does something different with it than what happens in human relationships. Transference in analysis is something problematic (that could even derail the treatment) that does not necessarily help the treatment. If anything, and as Winnicott pointed out, the analyst must survive the transference. This is clearly not the case with work transference within an organization although there can be a residue or transference work at work within work transference that threatens a psychoanalytic organization from within. Many personal transferences get acted out in the work of the organization as a communal structure and alleged democratic institution.

Traditionally, psychoanalytic institutions had guaranteed the transmission of their work, which in this case refers both to how psychoanalytic knowledge is being passed on generally, as well as to how new psychoanalysts are being trained, via a strict set of rules and regulations, controlled by an "executive board", which sits at the top of the institutional hierarchy. Possibly inspired by what he had observed in England during the Autumn of 1945 and emboldened by what he himself had experienced in his tumultuous relations with representatives of the SPP and the IPA, Lacan decided to organize his own School in a radically different way, although for many of its members this would prove to be an unfeasible, potentially deleterious initiative.

Dissolution

Working from the basic axiom that a psychoanalytic institution cannot function without psychoanalysts, Lacan came up with the provocative claim that a psychoanalyst derives his authorization only from himself (*le psychanalyste ne s'autorise que de lui-même*) (Lacan, 1995 [1967], p. 1), by which he meant that only someone's own analytic experience, i.e. the analysis that someone has undertaken, can equip him or her with the necessary "qualifications" to practice psychoanalytically, and not the successful completion of a "pseudo-academic" training programme, let alone the endorsement by an institutional hierarchy.

Although many people (mis)interpreted this principle as Lacan effectively suggesting that anyone should have the right to call himself a psychoanalyst—with potentially disastrous consequences for the clinical standards, the public image and the future of the discipline—in practice he argued in favour of the recognition of one single criterion for evaluating whether someone could be considered a psychoanalyst, and be authorized to practice: the personal experience of having been through the process of psychoanalysis.

Nonetheless, when presenting this principle to the EFP in October 1967, Lacan also considered the possibility of the School formally recognizing that someone had effectively been trained as a psychoanalyst and was working psychoanalytically, whereby he outlined two avenues for this recognition. First, the School may decide to bestow the title of "Analyst Member of the School" (AME) upon those practicing psychoanalysts who have demonstrated their analytic ability, in whatever form, and without the psychoanalysts themselves asking for this recognition. Second, analytic trainees and practicing analysts may themselves ask for institutional recognition, in which case they are required to speak about their own psychoanalytic journey, individually and independently, to three "passers"—members of the School who are roughly at the same point of their own trajectory and therefore "equals"—who subsequently transmit what they have heard to a decision-making body (the so-called "cartel of the pass"), which then deliberates as to whether the candidate should be given the title of "Analyst of the School" (AE) (Lacan, 1995 [1967], p. 1).

Lacan made it clear that these titles should not be interpreted in a hierarchical way, as the AMEs being superior to the AEs, or vice versa, but simply as different "steps" (*gradus*), each with their own duties and responsibilities. At the same time, he also reduced the power traditionally accorded to the training analyst, since he no longer wished to differentiate between a training analysis and a "regular analysis". Lacan did not see the need for potential analytic trainees to be treated differently from "normal patients" and did not want the training analysts to have the power to decide, or even to advise on how and when trainees should be recognized as psychoanalysts. In this non-hierarchical structure, and the radical decentralization of institutional power that Lacan attempted to bring about, here, we can once again detect an echo of Bion's ground-breaking experiments with leaderless groups.

The recruitment and selection of new psychoanalysts was not left to people in a position of authority, but candidates were able to self-select, insofar as they simply draw on their own analytic experience to apply their skills, demonstrate their capacity or satisfy independent observers. Much like the selection panel had operated in Bion's leaderless group experiments, the actual decision-making body does not evaluate the candidates directly but relies for its judgment on a set of non-partisans "witness statements". What matters is not whether someone has passed a requisite number of tests with flying colours—say a portfolio of examinations and coursework and the minimum amount of analytic sessions with a training analyst—but whether someone's subjective analytic experience shows sufficient clinical promise for that person to practice psychoanalytically.

So, did it all work? Because Lacan decided to dissolve his own School some fifteen years after it was created, one may be tempted to respond with a resounding "no". However, much like the Stalinist atrocities may not in themselves be a sufficient reason for confirming the intrinsic failure of the great communist experiment, Lacan's dissolution of the EFP may not as such be a reliable indicator of the fact that the entire organizational edifice was built on extremely loose foundations.

Despite Lacan's well-meaning attempt to diffuse institutional power, the EFP did not live up to the grand expectations that were raised on the day of its first inception. In transforming traditional hierarchical patters of operation into a "circular organization", Lacan was firmly convinced that the work of the School could be accomplished, and that doctrinal inertia could be averted, yet the institutional "consistency" that he believed would come with experience did not materialize, or gradually transformed itself again into a more conventional series of arrangements, with teachers and pupils, thinkers and disciples, leaders and followers, masters and servants.

The problem, no doubt, was to a large extent Lacan himself, who would always be the superior "plus one", the one who would not only stand out from the others because having been the one to found the

School (and therefore also being the only one who could subsequently legitimately disband it), but the one who was de facto intellectually unassailable, clinically infallible, institutionally unimpeachable.

Much like Bion in his Northfield experiments, Lacan recognized that the School expected him to demonstrate his authority as the leader of the organization in his capacity of Director of the School. Much like Bion, he accepted this responsibility, without therefore always complying with what the group was expecting of him. Yet this position of "suspended leadership", which constitutes an alternative position of agency—closer to that operating within the discourse of the analyst than that which is at work in the discourse of the master, following the distribution of functions in Lacan's famous "theory of the four discourses" (Lacan, 2007 [1969–1970]—gradually changed into a new, uncritical attribution of power.

Lacan's innovative mechanism for securing the institutional recognition of psychoanalysts who wish to be recognized as such, which came to be known as the "procedure of the pass", gradually showed its fractures. Witnesses were not believed to be as non-partisan and independent as could be hoped for. Testimonials were believed to be contaminated by the witnesses' knowledge of the identity of the candidates' own psychoanalysts. New artificial hierarchies started to emerge, and the work transference did not always manifest itself as creatively and productively as Lacan had wished for.

In a letter of 5 January 1980, Lacan announced that the School he had created some fifteen years earlier would be dissolved (Lacan, 1990 [1980]). One could no doubt see Lacan's decision, here, as an act of despair or frustration, or as an act signalling his own admission of organizational failure, yet one could also interpret it in a different light, as the intentional initiation of necessary transformational change. In the opening paragraphs of his letter, Lacan reminded his readership of the main reasons as to why he had decided to create the EFP: "[F]or a labor [...] which in the field opened by Freud restores the cutting edge of his truth—which brings the original praxis he instituted under the name of psychoanalysis back to the duty incumbent upon it in our world—which, through assiduous critique, denounces the deviations and compromises blunting its progress while degrading its use" (ibid.: 129). Hence, the dissolution of the organisation is a necessary precondition for the work towards the accomplishment of the primary task to be sustained. For the "circular organization" to survive, it must occasionally be dissolved and re-created, especially at a time when it seems to have reached a standstill, and when the members may be least expecting (or wanting) it, owing to the installation of a certain professional and socio-intellectual comfort.

Like the work-group that is the cartel, the "circular organization" has its life-span and must be disbanded, permutated and re-constructed to sustain itself as such. On 11 March 1980, towards the end of his last public seminar, Lacan invited the former members of his School to mourn, which also constitutes a kind of work, the death of their institutional home, and to become "de-Schooled" and "de-glued" (*d'écolé*), whilst at the same time announcing that a new organizational structure would be created, with the same structure of small working groups at its basis (Lacan, 1982 [1980], p. 87). If the *esprit de corps*, had been adversely affected by the work transference and enactments of transference work within the organization, this necessitated the dissolution of the School, and no dissolution should stand in the way of the re-creation of a new *esprit de corps*.

The Viability and Future of the Lacanian School as a Psychoanalytic Organization

As a theorist critical of psychoanalytic institutions, Lacan occupied himself with the recruitment and selection of candidates (for psychoanalytic formation), with the way in which (psychoanalytic) formation is delivered and monitored, with how the end of the formation process should be conceived, with how candidates who have finished their training should be recognized institutionally, and with typical "managerial" processes of (analytic) appraisal, evaluation and promotion. He was concerned about the stratification, the hierarchical structure, the allocation of authority, the distribution of power and the function of leadership in (psychoanalytic) institutions. He was deeply involved in setting the parameters for assuring institutional quality and standards, guaranteeing the organization's normative primary task, and securing its social and epistemological sustainability.

Despite Lacan's critique of the organizational structure of psychoanalytic institutions, and despite following Bion's experience with leaderless work groups and having the leader function in a state of suspended authority (an organizational model that Bion did not apply to the British Psychoanalytic Society), Lacan's reformations never completely deviated from the three functions that Eitingon (1922–1925) originally assigned to a psychoanalytic clinic: therapeutic, formative, and research. Lacan's school formed psychoanalysts, practiced psychoanalysis, and engaged in research and publication of written work.

In addition, in the Founding Act of his school Lacan emphasized denouncing the deviations and compromises that blunt and degrade psychoanalysis. This aim is not that different from the aim outlined by the International Psychoanalytic Conference of 1925 that

> sought to prevent the premature amalgamation and synthesis of psychoanalysis with other fields, research methods, and clinical practices. Given Freud's several initial problems with students who dissented/deviated from his teaching, the early international psychoanalytic movement was concerned with preserving and preventing the destruction of Freud's theory and practice. (idem, p. 223)

Moreover,

> The process of increased institutionalization and standardization of authority within psychoanalysis generated criticisms and questioning from the very beginning. Hans Sachs (Safouan, 1995) pointed out that wherever there is organization and hierarchy, the discovery of the new, and the possibility of change and transformation, becomes suppressed and repressed. Every institution is conservative in nature, and aims at its own survival and self-preservation and, therefore, has low tolerance for creative and inventive minds and subjects. (Moncayo, 2008, p. 224)

This would certainly apply to Lacan as an outstandingly creative and inventive psychoanalyst who thought that hierarchy and standardization was blunting the creative edge of psychoanalysis. Nevertheless, it remains unclear whether Lacan's organization succeeded in replacing traditional hierarchies, since even in the Pass procedure, the 'passers' introduced their own distortions to what was heard from the analysand and eventually a committee of analysts of the school decided whether a proper analysis had taken place. So, the hierarchy was maintained and produced two different class of analysts: those who passed the pass and those who did not but are still practicing analysts. Obviously given the structure of the organization, analysands would tend to choose analysts from those who had passed the pass.

Although the personal analysis is the necessary bedrock of analytic training, the question remains whether the personal analysis is sufficient criterion for the formation of psychoanalysts. A psychoanalyst of the school serves the public by offering psychoanalysis to those Lacan calls 'Little Shoes,' but a psychoanalytic organization requires candidates who enter the school to become psychoanalysts and need a personal analysis as part of this process (the Truly Necessary for the school).

However, Lacan always emphasized that a didactic analysis for purposes of formation was always a personal analysis like any other. In fact, an applicant should not be accepted into formation if they cannot present a symptom for analysis and instead view a personal analysis as a didactic process to learn the theory and practice of analysis (The Truly Necessary must be Little Shoes first).

At the Lacanian School of Psychoanalysis of the San Francisco Bay Area we followed Safouan (an early student of Lacan) in continuing the practice of control analysis or supervision as a necessary component of analytical formation (Safouan, 2000). Control analysis is second in importance but is not a replacement for the personal analysis. Lacan was concerned that the regulated supervision of the practice of analysis could become an organized resistance to the personal analysis and the work with the unconscious.

> During the 1974 Rome Congress of the *E.F.P.* (the Freudian School of Psychoanalysis), a consensus was building in the Lacanian field that, supervision, as a bureaucratic requirement, institutionalizes a resistance to analysis. Supervision, as an institutional requirement of so many certified years and hours, functions as an obsessional defense against dealing with difficulties inherent to the practice of analysis and the field of transference. Lacan believed that obligations with regards to the position of

> the analyst exempt or excuse a subject from the personal responsibility of having decided to do or not to do something. (idem, p. 29)

LSP made an early decision to require that analysts adhere to the licensing laws of California for the various professions. A license is the product of an alliance between the master's discourse or the discourse of government and the university discourse used to regulate government, business, and professional practice. A license does not authorize an analyst to practice psychoanalysis. In fact, since licenses do not require a personal analysis, all the regulations involving supervised experience miss the boat as to what guarantees best results for a member of the public benefitting from psychoanalysis.

When people approached Lacan for control he would refer them to analysis. Of course, this can vary if the person is a candidate of the school or the person already is in analysis or already had an analysis. The point here is that analysis is the first principle of formation, not that it's the only one.

There are forms of professional and even psychoanalytic practice for which formation does not require a personal analysis. An example would be the practice of psychoanalytic psychotherapy where supervision, for example, becomes an analysis of the countertransference as projective identification from the analysand to the analyst.

The point is not to critique various professional perspectives, but rather to understand, in our current context, how Lacan may have been responding to a demand for supervision as a demand for analysis or even as a resistance to analysis.

In any case, what is a control analysis or supervision of psychoanalysis (to use arbitrary semantic terms for a moment without delving too much into the limitations of their literal meanings)? Supervision has always existed alongside the personal analysis in psychoanalytic institutions, sometimes with the same analyst but more likely with two different analysts. As we shall see, control and supervision are both arbitrary deficient terms to describe an analytical state of suspended authority. A control analyst neither controls nor has 'super-vision' like superman. If anything, control analysis is a form of 'other-audition': what the analyst hears in what the analyst heard of the analysand's speech that the candidate analyst does not know that they know. This is what Reik (1998) called listening with the Third ear. The Third is the place where the sense organ and the object of sound meet *savoir* or unconscious knowing or a form of un-self-conscious-knowledge (a form of subjective objectivity).

The control analyst also helps a candidate analyst articulate or put into use the theory in relationship to the practice of analysis. In addition, it is also implied that a candidate analyst participates in seminars, case conferences, and the study of psychoanalytic theory and practice as fundamental aspects of analytical formation.

These two practices (personal and control analysis) plus the study of the theory constitute the triptic of psychoanalytic education and formation. But ultimately for Lacan the analyst is authorized by their own symptom become *sinthome* in life and the personal analysis. At the same time the entire organization stands on the subject's desire as the motivating factor. At LSP candidates have a responsibility to keep the record of what they have done by way of meeting the requirements of the School. The record is a testament to their desire for analysis and professional formation. This minimizes the bureaucratic dimension and at the same time prevents that formation simply become a demand of the Other, or a discourse of the master, or the discourse of the university.

Although Lacan declared that the Pass procedure had failed

> Lacan never gave up the idea of the privileged role of the personal analysis for the practice of analysis but he did give up trying to evaluate it in any kind of institutional or objective fashion. Instead he turned his attention to the theoretical question of the *sinthome* as what ultimately authorizes an analyst. (idem, p. 31)

However, although standarization or objective evaluation of analysis is ultimately impossible, there are criteria by which to determine if an analysis is taking place in the proper sense of the term. For example, with regards to the transference to the 'subject supposed to know' (*sujet suppose savoir*) two things need to take place: (1) A positive transference needs to established; (2) The analyst has to remove himself/herself from the position of the 'subject supposed to know' without losing the positive transference that allows the Ucs. of the analysand to manifest.

When the positive transference is established the analyst says very little to the analysand and approves most of what they say, except in extraordinary circumstances, of course. The analyst accepts the defenses that the ego uses to describe their problems and hears the saying that emerges in the space between words and within the narrative statement (the said).

The positive transference cannot be described as a desire of the analyst to be liked because otherwise this would be transference and something that the analyst had to work out in his/her own analysis. In fact, the desire of the analyst not to be idealized in the transference supports the strength of the positive transference and can be considered a fruit of the personal analysis. The positive transference is not a response to the desire to be liked and loved but rather to a strategy of *savoir* and a question of correct method. The desire to be liked and admired is a characteristic of the histerical master in the formula for the master's discourse: $\frac{S_1}{\$} \rightarrow \frac{S_2}{a}$. The master's lack demands that subjects/servants locate the *objet a* in them.

The social organizational consequence of the first criterion to carry out or evaluate an analysis, is that the analyst accepts the leadership of the position but then uses it in a different way. This different use is the relinquishing of the position of SsS, a veritable symbolic castration of the position of the master that transforms the position from a master position to an analytical position. This is the democratic principle that Lacan envisioned. A free association that permits the Unconscious or the unconscious signifying chain and the Real to emerge. The analyst is an S_0 instead of the S_1 of the master. The S_0 is the *objet a* in the place of the agent in the formula for the analyst's discourse. The analyst moves from the position of the beloved imaginary object (*a*/phallus), to the position of the absence or emptiness of the *objet a*.

But what authorizes an analyst? Lacan (1995 [1967]) famously stated that the analyst is authorized by himself/herself and then he added and a few others. What does this mean? It does not mean that an analyst is self-taught and self-appointed as an analyst without any psychoanalytic formation or association to a Lacanian school. From this point of view self-authorization on the basis of a personal analysis alone or on the basis of a professional degree or license could be equally problematic.

Sometimes people may combine these elements on their own (including attendance to seminars or study groups) in which cases a school may accept those analysts (as well as others trained in other analytic organizations) as Analysts Member of the School so long as they support the School and its principles. The Analyst of the School is still necessary since the reference to the barred Other of the school allows for the transmission and articulation of the triptic of analytical formation (analysis, control, and *savoir*). However, at LSP we have eliminated the category of Beatitudes or Training Analysts chosen by their peers and any Analyst of the School can be chosen by a candidate as a supervising or control analyst.

An analyst is authorized by the desire that drives their formation rather than by the requirements of an institution. The others of a school are merely witnesses of the work the candidate analyst has accomplished. At LSP the analyst in formation is responsible to keep the record of how they have fulfilled the requirements of the school. Formation begins with a declaration to others of the subject's desire to be a psychoanalyst (what is called a Palimpsest) and concludes with a statement of their desire, on the basis of a record, to finish their formation. What we call the 'Passage', is the act of presenting a paper or case to the community and assume the name of Analyst of the School (an act of Nomination, therefore). In addition, they may speak to an analyst outside the school about their personal experience of the Unconscious in analysis.

At LSP we encourage candidates not only to participate in seminars but also to lead seminars in a state of suspended authority. This notion of suspended authority here means two things: (1) That the seminar leader shares the teaching seat with participants; and (2) That leading a seminar does not mean that the leader no longer takes seminars led by other analysts/candidates/faculty of the school. One of the potential pitfalls of this model is that a seminar may become a fiefdom/chiefdom or a way for the candidate to ascend through the ranks of the organization.

On the other hand, the school is not without the consequences of a meritocracy on the basis of the candidates own scholarly work and research as an end in itself. The analyst, more than being identified with a profession or with the name and gain associated with professional expertise, is a metaphor for the subject who knows about non knowing and unconscious knowing. In addition, by the same token that the analyst suspends the position or attitude of the master, a psychoanalytic school needs to be open and receptive to inborn and cultivated talent without invidious comparison to others. Such talent builds the reservoir of *savoir* of a school which is what Lacan was able to accomplish while running the risk of becoming the only voice and text of the school.

It should not be the sole responsibility of one single individual to create or dissolve a school. In addition, it is important to differentiate between constructive and destructive/nihilistic forms of emptying out or dissolving/changing a structure. As argued in previous chapters, structures are already empty, and are only reified by the impregnations of the ego, the master, and the Imaginary. The 'few others' of authorization represent the necessity of a demystified and barred Other (not a master institution) to function as a guarantee of the psychoanalytic organization as an open system subject to change and evolution, both positive and negative. This criterion may be more important than thinking that all organizations should be periodically dissolved and reinvented. In fact, Lacan's dissolution of his school, led to the establishment of a new organization that according to some has become even more undemocratic than the IPA. In addition, many alternative Lacanian organizations have sprung up that continue to exist to this day without being dissolved by their founders.

Finally, what is the difference between a study group, a cartel, a seminar, and a work group. Which one is a work group in the sense that Bion meant it? A study group can be a leaderless group but often has a leader that comments and expounds on a text being read. The cartel with the plus one is a way to combine both factors except that the plus one does not teach but rather assigns and coordinates the work tasks of the group. A cartel does not resolve the problem of the difference in talent and motivational desire among members of a group.

Leadership may still emerge within a group since a school is the work and talent that members bring to the school. However, talent here is not resolved in the direction of artificial intelligence or the intellectual power of computation and information within a binary system (like a robot or automaton who wants to be smarter than people or other people). Talent ends in *savoir* or a form of unknown knowing (*l'insu qui sait*) that cancels out the ego ideal of the master and points rather to the human subject of the Real that responds to and follows from Tyche and Nous rather than automaton or a robot of instrumental/technical reason.

A seminar allows for the leadership of talent and effort while at the same time being a work group in the sense that the leader as an analyst functions as S_0 in a state of suspended (ego master) authority and shares the teaching seat with participants who can also present their work. In the work group, Bion accepted the leadership bestowed upon him by his own work and the group but used it in a different way according to a category of reason known as *savoir* in Lacan and knowing of O in Bion. The latter continues a tradition of mind in Western philosophy known as Nous from the pre-Socratics, through Aristotle, to Husserl's phenomenology and Heidegger, and the Frankfurt School. This transmission of mind is absent in the master's discourse and the university discourse and remains alive in the analytic tradition invented/discovered by Freud.

References

Arnaud, G. (2002). The Organization and the Symbolic: Organizational Dynamics Viewed from a Lacanian Perspective. *Human Relations, 55*, 691–716.

Arnaud, G. (2003). A Coach or a Couch? A Lacanian Perspective on Executive Coaching and Consulting. *Human Relations, 56*, 1131–1154.

Arnaud, G., & Vanheule, S. (2007). The Division of the Subject and the Organization: A Lacanian Approach to Subjectivity at Work. *Journal of Organizational Change Management, 20*, 359–369.

Beattie, T. (2013). *Theology After Postmodernity: Divining the Void–A Lacanian Reading of Thomas Aquinas*. Oxford and New York, NY: Oxford University Press.

Bicknell, M., & Liefooghe, A. (2010). Enjoy Your Stress! Using Lacan to Enrich Transactional Models of Stress. *Organization, 17*, 317–330.

Bion, W. R. (1946). Leaderless Group Project. *Bulletin of the Menninger Clinic, 10*, 77–81.

Bion, W. R. (1961 [1948–1951]). Experiences in Groups. In *Experiences in Groups and Other Papers* (pp. 27–137). London: Routledge.

Bion, W. R. (1961 [1952]). Group Dynamics. In *Experiences in Groups and Other Papers* (pp. 139–191). London: Routledge.

Bloom, P., & Cederström, D. (2009). The Sky's the Limit: Fantasy in the Age of Market Rationality. *Journal of Organizational Change Management, 22,* 159–180.

Caudill, D. S. (1997). *Lacan and the Subject of Law: Toward a Psychoanalytic Critical Legal Theory*. Atlantic Highlands, NJ: Humanities Press.

Cho, K. D. (2009). *Psychopedagogy: Freud, Lacan, and the Psychoanalytic Theory of Education*. Basingstoke and New York, NY: Palgrave Macmillan.

Costas, J., & Taheri, A. (2012). 'The Return of the Primal Father' in Postmodernity? A Lacanian Analysis of Authentic Leadership. *Organization Studies, 33,* 1195–1216.

Driver, M. (2009a). From Loss to Lack: Stories of Organizational Change as Encounters with Failed Fantasies of Self, Work and Organization. *Organization, 16,* 353–369.

Driver, M. (2009b). Struggling with Lack: A Lacanian Perspective on Organizational Identity. *Organization Studies, 30,* 55–72.

Driver, M. (2009c). Encountering the Arugula Leaf: The Failure of the Imaginary and Its Implications for Research on Identity in Organizations. *Organization, 16,* 487–504.

Driver, M. (2014). The Stressed Subject: Lack, Empowerment and Liberation. *Organization, 21,* 90–105.

Eissler, R. S. (1954). 106th Bulletin of the International Psycho-analytical Association. *The International Journal of Psycho-analysis, 35,* 267–290.

Etchegoyen, R. H., & Miller, J. A. (1996). *Silence brisé. Entretien sur le mouvement psychanalytique*. Paris: Agalma.

Fotaki, M. (2009). Maintaining the Illusion of a Free Health Service in Post-socialism: A Lacanian Analysis of Transition from Planned to Market Economy. *Journal of Organizational Change Management, 22,* 141–158.

Freud, S. (1914). Remembering, Repeating and Working-Through (Further Recommendations on the Technique of Psycho-analysis II). SE, XII, 145–156.

Glynos, J. (2011). On the Ideological and Political Significance of Fantasy in the Organization of Work. *Psychoanalysis, Culture and Society, 16,* 373–393.

Harding, N. (2007). On Lacan and the Becoming-ness of Organizations/Selves. *Organization Studies, 28,* 1761–1773.

Harrison, T. (2000). *Bion, Rickman, Foulkes and the Northfield Experiments: Advancing on a Different Front*. London: Jessica Kingsley.
Hendrix, J. S. (2006). *Architecture and Psychoanalysis: Peter Eisenman and Jacques Lacan*. New York, NY: Peter Lang.
Jagodzinski, J. (2005). *Music in Youth Culture: A Lacanian Approach*. Basingstoke and New York, NY: Palgrave Macmillan.
Johnsen, R., & Gudmand-Høyer, M. (2010). Lacan and the Lack of Humanity in HRM. *Organization, 17*, 331–344.
Jones, C., & Spicer, A. (2005). The Sublime Object of Entrepreneurship. *Organization, 12*, 223–246.
Kenny, K. (2009). Heeding the Stains: Lacan and Organizational Change. *Journal of Organizational Change Management, 22*, 214–228.
Kosmala, K., & Herrbach, O. (2006). The Ambivalence of Professional Identity: On Cynicism and Jouissance in Audit Firms. *Human Relations, 59*, 1393–1428.
Lacan, J. (1968). Proposition du 9 Octobre sur la psychanalyse a l'Ecole. *Scilicet, 1*, 14–30.
Lacan, J. (1976 [1949]). Règlement et doctrine de la commission de l'enseignement. In J.-A. Miller (Ed.), *La scission de 1953. La communauté psychanalytique en France I* (pp. 29–36). Paris: Navarin.
Lacan, J. (1976 [1975]). Interventions dans la séance de travail sur 'Du plus une'. *Lettres de l'École freudienne, 18*, 219–229.
Lacan, J. (1982 [1980]). D'écolage. *École de la cause freudienne–Annuaire et textes statutaires*. Paris: ECF.
Lacan, J. (1988 [1953–1954]). *The Seminar, Book I, Freud's Papers on Technique* (J.-A. Miller, Ed., J. Forrester, Trans.). Cambridge: Cambridge University Press.
Lacan, J. (1990 [1963]). Introduction to the Names-of-the-Father Seminar. In J. Copjec (Ed.), *Television/A Challenge to the Psychoanalytic Establishment* (J. Mehlman, Trans., pp. 81–95). New York, NY: W.W. Norton.
Lacan, J. (1990 [1964]). Founding Act. In J. Copjec (Ed.), *Television/A Challenge to the Psychoanalytic Establishment* (J. Mehlman, Trans., pp. 97–106). New York, NY: W.W. Norton.
Lacan, J. (1990 [1980]). Letter of Dissolution. In J. Copjec (Ed.), *Television/A Challenge to the Psychoanalytic Establishment* (J. Mehlman, Trans., pp. 129–131). New York, NY: W.W. Norton.
Lacan, J. (1994 [1964]). *The Seminar, Book XI, the Four Fundamental Concepts of Psychoanalysis* (J.-A. Miller, Ed., A. Sheridan, Trans.). Harmondsworth: Penguin.

Lacan, J. (1995 [1967]). Proposition of 9 October 1967 on the Psychoanalyst of the School (R. Grigg, Trans.). *Analysis, 6*, 1–13.

Lacan, J. (2000 [1947]). British Psychiatry and the War (P. Dravers & V. Voruz, Trans.). *Psychoanalytical Notebooks of the London Circle, 4*, 9–33.

Lacan, J. (2006 [1953]). The Function and Field of Speech and Language in Psychoanalysis. In *Écrits* (B. Fink, Trans., pp. 197–268). New York, NY and London: W.W. Norton.

Lacan, J. (2006 [1956]). The Situation of Psychoanalysis and the Training of Psychoanalysts in 1956. In *Écrits* (B. Fink, Trans., pp. 384–411). New York, NY and London: W.W. Norton.

Lacan, J. (2006 [1958]). The Direction of the Treatment and the Principles of Its Power. In *Écrits* (B. Fink, Trans., pp. 489–542). New York, NY and London: W.W. Norton.

Lacan, J. (2006 [1962]). Kant with Sade. In *Écrits* (B. Fink, Trans., pp. 645–668). New York, NY and London: W.W. Norton.

Lacan, J. (2006 [1968–1969]). *Le Séminaire, Livre XVI, D'un Autre à l'autre*, texte établi par J.-A. Miller. Paris: du Seuil.

Lacan, J. (2007 [1969–1970]). *The Seminar, Book XVII, the Other Side of Psychoanalysis* (J.-A. Miller, Ed., R. Grigg, Trans.). New York, NY and London: W.W. Norton.

Lacan, J. (2014 [1962–1963]). *The Seminar, Book X, Anxiety* (J.-A. Miller, Ed., A. Price, Trans.). Cambridge: Polity.

Miller, J. A. (Ed.). (1976). *La scission de 1953. La communauté psychanalytique en France I*. Paris: Navarin.

Miller, J. A. (Ed.). (1977). *L'excommunication. La communauté psychanalytique en France II*. Paris: Navarin.

Miller, P. A. (2007). *Postmodern Spiritual Practices: The Construction of the Subject and the Reception of Plato in Lacan, Derrida, and Foucault*. Columbus, OH: Ohio State University Press.

Milovanovic, D. (2003). *Critical Criminology at the Edge: Postmodern Perspectives, Integration, and Applications*. Boulder, CO: Lynne Rienner.

Moncayo, R. (2008). *Evolving Lacanian Perspectives for Clinical Psychoanalysis: On Narcissism, Sexuation, and the Phases of Analysis in Contemporary Culture*. London: Karnac Books.

Nobus, D. (2016). Esprit de corps, Work Transference and Dissolution: Lacan as an Organizational Theorist. *Psychoanalytische Perspectieven, 34*(4), 355–378.

Reik, T. (1998 [1948]). *Listening with the Third Ear*. New York: Farrar, Straus and Giroux.

Roudinesco, E. (1997 [1993]). *Jacques Lacan* (B. Bray, Trans.). New York, NY and London: Columbia University Press.
Safouan, M. (2000). *Jacques Lacan and the Question of Psychoanalytic Training*. London: Macmillan.
Stavrakakis, Y. (2008). Subjectivity and the Organized Other: Between Symbolic Authority and Fantasmatic Enjoyment. *Organization Studies, 29*, 1037–1059.
Turquet, P. (2014). *Le rapport Turquet* (L. Parisel, Trans.). Paris: Cahiers de l'Unebévue.
Van Haute, Ph. (2002 [2000]). *Against Adaptation: Lacan's 'Subversion of the Subject'—A Close Reading* (P. Crowe & M. Vankerk, Trans.). New York, NY: Other Press.
Vanheule, S., Lievrouw, A., & Verhaeghe, P. (2003). Burnout and Intersubjectivity: A Psychoanalytical Study from a Lacanian Perspective. *Human Relations, 56*, 321–338.
Vanheule, S., & Verhaeghe, P. (2004). Powerlessness and Impossibility in Special Education: A Qualitative Study on Professional Burnout from a Lacanian Perspective. *Human Relations, 57*, 497–519.
Vidaillet, B. (2007). Lacanian Theory's Contribution to the Study of Workplace Envy. *Human Relations, 60*, 1669–1700.
Vidaillet, B., & Gamot, G. (2015). Working and Resisting When One's Workplace Is Under Threat of Being Shut Down: A Lacanian Perspective. *Organization Studies, 36*, 987–1011.

Index

R. Moncayo, *Knowing, Not-Knowing, and Jouissance*, The Palgrave Lacan Series,
https://doi.org/10.1007/978-3-319-94003-8

N

O

P

Z

FSC
www.fsc.org
MIX
Papier | Fördert
gute Waldnutzung
FSC® C083411

Kolibri 360 GmbH
Ferdinand-Jühlke-Straße 7
99095 Erfurt, Deutschland
produktsicherheit@kolibri360.de